The New Atkins Diet for Beginners 2025

Transform Your Body, Change Your Life with These Easy and Effective Low-Carb Strategies

Protein Pg.59

By

DAPHNE S. ABSHER

About The Author

Daphne S. Absher is a passionate advocate for healthy living and a dedicated nutrition enthusiast with a deep understanding of low-carb lifestyles. With years of personal experience and extensive research in the field of nutrition, Daphne has transformed her own health journey and aims to inspire others to achieve their wellness goals. Her engaging writing style and commitment to empowering readers make her an invaluable resource for those looking to embrace a healthier way of eating.

Daphne believes that food is not just a source of nourishment, but a means to enhance overall well-being and vitality. Through her work, she seeks to demystify the complexities of nutrition, providing practical advice and easy-to-follow strategies that fit into busy lives. She is dedicated to sharing the latest insights and research in the ever-evolving world of low-carb diets, ensuring her readers have access to the most effective tools and resources.

Daphne loves experimenting in the kitchen, creating delicious and satisfying low-carb recipes that everyone can enjoy. She believes that healthy eating should never be boring, and her culinary creations reflect that philosophy.

Daphne invites you to join her on this exciting journey toward better health and wellness. Be sure to check out her other books for more tips, recipes, and strategies to enhance your weight loss lifestyle. If you found this book helpful, feel free to recommend it to friends and loved ones. Together, you can inspire each other to live healthier, happier lives!

NEW EDITION

THE NEW ATKINS DIET

FOR BEGINNERS

2025

ADDED BONUS

TRANSFORM YOUR BODY, CHANGE YOUR LIFE WITH THESE EASY AND EFFECTIVE LOW-CARB STRATEGIES

165 LOW-CARB SHOPPING LIST IDEAS

DAPHNE S. ABSHER

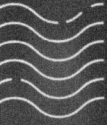

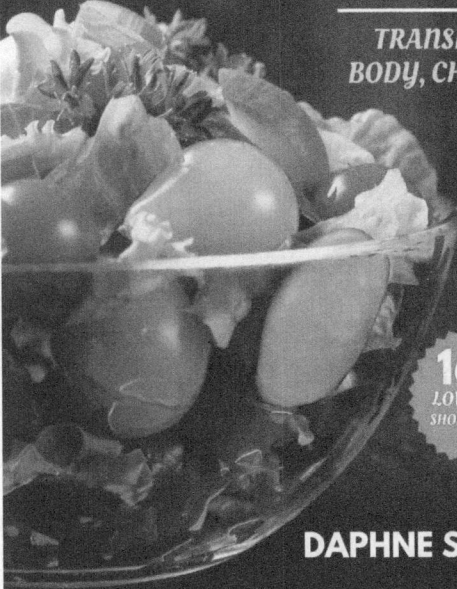

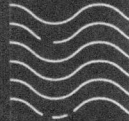

Table of contents

INTRODUCTION

Welcome to the New Atkins Diet, a revolutionary approach to weight loss and optimal health. For decades, the Atkins Diet has been a household name, synonymous with effective and sustainable weight management. This updated edition incorporates the latest scientific research, nutritional insights, and practical strategies to help you achieve your goals.

The Atkins Diet's core principle remains unchanged: by restricting carbohydrate intake, you unlock your body's natural ability to burn fat for energy. This simple yet powerful concept has transformed the lives of millions worldwide. By embracing a low-carb lifestyle, you'll not only shed unwanted pounds but also experience improved blood sugar control, enhanced energy levels, and reduced inflammation.

So, what sets the New Atkins Diet apart from other weight loss plans? Its flexible and adaptable approach recognizes that every individual is unique, with distinct nutritional needs and lifestyle preferences. Rather than imposing unrealistic restrictions or cookie-cutter meal plans, the New Atkins Diet empowers you to make informed choices, gradually introducing healthier habits into your daily routine.

At its heart, the New Atkins Diet is a holistic approach to wellness, encompassing nutrition, physical activity, and mental well-being. By focusing on whole, nutrient-dense foods, you'll nourish your body and satisfy your appetite. Fresh vegetables, lean proteins, healthy fats, and whole grains form the foundation of your new eating habits.

As you embark on this journey, you'll discover the freedom to enjoy your favorite foods in moderation, without guilt or deprivation. This book isn't a quick fix or a fad; it's a sustainable lifestyle transformation. By making conscious choices, you'll develop a deeper understanding of your body's needs and cultivate a positive relationship with food.

Recent studies have reaffirmed the effectiveness of low-carb diets for weight loss and improved metabolic health. Research published in the Journal of the American Medical Association and the American Journal of Clinical Nutrition demonstrates the significant benefits of restricting carbohydrate intake.

As you begin your journey, remember that every small step counts. The New Atkins Diet For Beginners 2025 is more than a weight loss plan – it's a path to vibrant health, increased energy, and a renewed sense of purpose. Transform, thrive and discover a happier you.

Chapter 1: Welcome to the New Atkins Diet

Understanding the Basics

Starting a new way of eating can feel both exciting and overwhelming. You're stepping into something fresh, and with it comes the promise of change. The beauty of this approach lies in its simplicity: it's not about deprivation but about making mindful choices that work with your body, not against it. This journey is about embracing a shift in how you fuel yourself, and it's simpler than you might think.

The first thing to understand is that you're not diving into something extreme or complicated. It's really about focusing on eating real, whole foods while minimizing those that can work against your goals. You're not counting every bite or meticulously tracking every detail, but rather finding a sustainable rhythm that feels natural over time. It's about knowing which foods give you energy and which ones hold you back.

This approach is built around reducing certain things that often sneak into everyday meals without us even noticing. These are the kinds of foods that might taste good in the moment but leave you feeling sluggish later on. When you begin to shift your focus to more nutrient-dense options, you'll quickly notice how much better you feel—not just physically, but mentally too. Energy levels rise, and you start feeling more in control.

One of the most freeing aspects of this shift is that it doesn't require perfection. Relax and enjoy your food, don't obsess over every bite. Instead, you'll be learning to make choices that align with your goals most of the time. The occasional indulgence isn't something to fear. What matters more is the overall pattern of your choices. And over time, these choices will become second nature.

The key to success is in the foundation. It starts with understanding how your body responds to the types of foods you eat. When you shift away from refined options and focus on real, satisfying ingredients, your body begins to operate more efficiently. Cravings that once seemed hard to ignore will diminish as you discover how satisfying these new meals can be. You'll be fuller for longer, feeling more satisfied with what you're eating.

Another important thing to keep in mind is that everyone's journey looks different. What works for one person might not be the exact fit for another. That's okay! There's no one-size-fits-all here. The goal is to find what feels good for you, which foods give you the energy you need, and how to build meals that you genuinely enjoy.

Remember, this isn't a quick fix but a lifestyle shift. Endure the short-term struggle for a lifetime of benefits. Once you understand the basics and start feeling the results, you'll realize that it's not about restriction, but rather about giving your body what it needs to thrive. As you get started, stay patient with yourself. Focus on progress, not perfection; every small win counts. Each choice you make is a step towards feeling better and being healthier.

The best part? You're in control of this journey. You get to decide what works for you, and the flexibility is part of what makes it so effective. Once you have a clear understanding of these basics, the rest will fall into place. You're setting yourself up for success—so enjoy the process, stay curious, and get ready to experience a new way of living that supports your best self.

The Science Behind Low-Carb Weight Loss

At first, it might seem surprising that simply changing the types of foods you eat can lead to significant weight loss. But there's a fascinating process that happens in the body when you reduce certain kinds of foods. It's all rooted in how your body uses energy. Every time you eat, your body decides how to turn that food into fuel. When you shift the balance of what you're eating, your body switches gears, tapping into a different and more efficient energy source. This switch is one of the key reasons why this approach works so well for many people, and it can lead to incredible results without constantly feeling hungry or deprived.

To understand how this works, let's start with the basics of how the body uses energy. Typically, when you eat, your body breaks down carbohydrates into sugars, which are used as a quick and easy source of energy. These sugars are sent into the bloodstream, where they power your activities throughout the day. However, when you reduce the intake of carbohydrates, your body doesn't have as much of that quick-burning fuel. Instead, it turns to stored energy reserves as a backup source. This is where the magic begins to happen. Your body becomes more efficient at burning stored energy, leading to a gradual but steady reduction in overall reserves.

This process is what makes this method so effective. Instead of constantly feeding on quick-burning energy from your meals, your body learns to tap into what's already stored inside. This switch isn't just about cutting back on food but about training your body to use energy differently. At first, this change might feel a little strange. Your body is used to getting quick energy from refined foods, and when that's no longer available, there might be an adjustment period. However, once this shift happens, your energy levels become much steadier, and the results start to show.

One of the reasons this approach works so well is because of how it impacts a key hormone responsible for regulating energy storage. This hormone plays a significant role in deciding whether your body uses energy for immediate fuel or stores it for later. When you eat a lot of refined foods, this hormone goes into overdrive, causing more energy to be stored rather than used. This is why many people find that their energy reserves increase over time, leading to frustration and difficulty reaching their goals. However, by reducing quick-energy sources, you give this hormone a chance to calm down and settle into a healthier balance. This, in turn, makes it easier for your body to manage energy effectively.

In addition to helping with energy storage, reducing certain foods has a profound impact on hunger levels and cravings. Many people are used to experiencing energy spikes and crashes throughout the day, especially after eating meals high in refined options. This pattern can lead to constant feelings of hunger or the need to snack regularly to maintain energy. However, when you switch to more nutrient-dense foods, you may find that you're fuller for longer periods and that cravings start to fade away. This happens because nutrient-dense foods provide more stable, long-lasting energy, helping you feel satisfied without the constant urge to snack.

Another important scientific aspect of this method is how it affects the body's metabolism. When you rely on quick-burning energy sources like refined foods, your body can become less efficient at using energy over time. However, when you encourage your body to use stored energy, it becomes better at converting those reserves into fuel. This is one reason why some people find that their energy levels actually improve after making this shift. Your body learns to rely on its reserves, and this leads to a more consistent level of energy throughout the day.

What's fascinating is how this approach isn't just about physical transformation but also mental and emotional shifts. When you rely less on quick-energy foods, you start to feel more in control of your cravings, and your mood can stabilize as well. Many people report feeling more balanced, less irritable, and more focused once their body adjusts to this shift. This happens because your energy is no longer spiking and crashing throughout the day.

It's important to understand that this method isn't forcing your body into anything unnatural. In fact, it's more aligned with how your body is designed to function. When you encourage your body to use energy from its reserves, you're allowing it to operate in a way that supports long-term health and balance. The science behind this process is well-researched, and it's been proven to be effective for many people. It's not a temporary fix but a way to help your body find a more natural, sustainable rhythm for managing energy.

As you continue on this journey, you'll notice that your body becomes more efficient at using its reserves for energy. This is a key reason why this approach has lasting power—it helps you build a system where your body isn't constantly dependent on what you eat right in the moment but instead uses what it already has. Over time, you'll see and feel the benefits of this, not just in your physical appearance but in how you feel day-to-day. The science behind this shift is powerful, and as you embrace it, you'll start to see just how effective it can be in helping you reach your goals, both physically and mentally.

Setting Your Weight Loss Goals and Expectations

Embarking on a weight loss journey is an exciting venture, but it's essential to set clear goals and realistic expectations to ensure success. The foundation of this journey lies in understanding what you want to achieve and how you can reach those milestones without overwhelming yourself. Each person's journey is unique, so take the time to define what success looks like for you.

First, it's important to establish specific, measurable goals. Rather than vague aspirations like "I want to lose weight," think in terms of concrete numbers and timelines. For example, setting a goal to lose a certain amount of weight within a specific time frame gives you a clear target to aim for. This doesn't mean you have to be rigid; rather, it allows you to track your progress and celebrate the small victories along the way. By breaking your larger goal into smaller milestones, you can create a sense of accomplishment as you reach each one, motivating you to keep going.

However, while it's vital to have goals, it's equally important to keep your expectations realistic. Weight loss can vary greatly from person to person due to various factors, including metabolism, activity level, and individual circumstances. It's natural for progress to ebb and flow. Instead of expecting to shed a large amount of weight every week, aim for a steady, gradual decrease. This not only makes the journey more manageable but also helps solidify new habits that will benefit you long after you've reached your target weight. Aiming for a pound or two each week is a realistic expectation for many people, but remember that some weeks may yield different results.

A strong mindset is the driving force behind reaching your objectives. Embrace a positive and flexible attitude. There will be days when you feel motivated and inspired, and there will be days when you face challenges. On those tough days, remember that setbacks are a natural part of any journey. Don't be disheartened - treat obstacles as catalysts for self improvement and refinement.

Another aspect of goal-setting is to consider the "why" behind your journey. Understanding your motivations will help keep you focused during challenging times. Whether it's to feel more energetic, improve your health, or boost your confidence, anchoring your goals for personal reasons can provide a deeper sense of purpose. Write down your motivations and revisit them regularly to remind yourself why you started this journey.

In addition to setting weight loss goals, it's beneficial to include non-scale victories in your expectations. These can include increased energy levels, improved sleep, better mood, or fitting into clothes that previously felt tight. Recognizing and celebrating these achievements can enhance your motivation and remind you that weight loss is not just about the number on the scale. It's about improving your overall well-being.

As you set your goals and expectations, consider creating a support system. Whether it's friends, family, or online communities, having a network of encouragement can make a world of difference. Sharing your goals with others can help keep you accountable and motivated. Plus, connecting with others on a similar journey can provide valuable insights, tips, and emotional support.

Finally, remember that your journey is personal and ongoing. Goals can evolve, and that's perfectly okay. As you progress, you may find new aspirations emerging or existing ones needing adjustment. Stay open to change and growth, and keep your focus on creating lasting, positive habits that contribute to your health and happiness. By setting thoughtful goals and maintaining realistic expectations, you'll be well-equipped to navigate your weight loss journey with confidence and determination.

Chapter 2: Preparing for Success

Understanding Macronutrients: Protein, Fat, and Carbohydrates

As you embark on your journey toward healthier living, understanding macronutrients is a vital step in preparing for success. These three essential components—protein, fat, and carbohydrates—are the building blocks of your diet. Each macronutrient plays a unique role in your body, and knowing how they work together can help you make informed choices that align with your goals.

Let's start with protein. Often hailed as the body's building block, protein is essential for growth, repair, and maintenance of tissues. When you consume protein, your body breaks it down into amino acids, which are then used to create new proteins needed for everything from muscle recovery to hormone production. Including adequate protein in your meals can also aid in weight management. It has a higher thermic effect compared to fats and carbohydrates, meaning your body burns more calories digesting protein than it does with the other two macronutrients. Additionally, protein is incredibly satiating, helping you feel fuller for longer periods. This can be particularly beneficial when you're trying to manage your appetite and reduce unnecessary snacking.

When selecting protein sources, consider a variety of options to ensure you get a broad spectrum of amino acids. Lean meats, poultry, fish, eggs, dairy products, legumes, and plant-based proteins like tofu and tempeh can all contribute to your protein intake. Aim to include protein in each meal, whether it's a hearty breakfast with eggs, a satisfying lunch with chicken salad, or a dinner featuring grilled fish. By making protein a priority, you set a strong foundation for your dietary success.

Next, let's explore fat. Once vilified in many diets, fat is now recognized as an essential component of a healthy eating plan. Fats play numerous roles in the body, including providing energy, supporting cell growth, and aiding in the absorption of fat-soluble vitamins such as A, D, E, and K. Additionally, healthy fats can contribute to heart health by reducing inflammation and improving cholesterol levels. Including a variety of fats in your diet can also help maintain stable blood sugar levels, which is especially important when you're trying to manage your weight.

Not all fats are created equal, so it's important to focus on incorporating healthy sources of fat into your meals. Monounsaturated fats, found in foods like avocados, olive oil, and nuts, are particularly beneficial. Omega-3 fatty acids, found in fatty fish such as salmon and flaxseeds, also offer impressive health benefits, including supporting brain function and reducing inflammation. On the other hand, it's wise to limit saturated and trans fats, which are often found in processed foods and can contribute to health issues when consumed in excess.

Lastly, let's discuss carbohydrates, often viewed with suspicion in many diets. Carbohydrates are a primary energy source for the body, fueling everything from daily activities to workouts. However, not all carbohydrates are equal. Refined carbohydrates, such as white bread, sugary snacks, and soft drinks, can lead to spikes in blood sugar levels and are often stripped of their natural nutrients. Instead, focusing on whole, unprocessed carbohydrates is key. These include whole grains, fruits, vegetables, and legumes, which provide fiber, vitamins, and minerals that support overall health.

Incorporating fiber-rich carbohydrates into your meals has additional benefits. Fiber not only helps regulate digestion but also aids in feelings of fullness. Foods high in fiber take longer to digest, which can help prevent those energy crashes and cravings that often accompany refined carbohydrate consumption. Consider adding foods like quinoa, brown rice, whole-grain bread, and a variety of fruits and vegetables to your plate. They not only offer essential nutrients but also contribute to overall satisfaction during meals.

As you prepare for success on your journey, consider how these three macronutrients can work together harmoniously. Strive for balance in your meals, aiming to include protein, healthy fats, and complex carbohydrates at each sitting. This balanced approach will not only help you meet your nutritional needs but will also keep your energy levels stable throughout the day.

Experimenting with different combinations can be enjoyable and can lead to discovering new favorite meals. For instance, a quinoa salad topped with grilled chicken, avocado, and a variety of colorful vegetables offers a delightful blend of all three macronutrients. Meanwhile, a breakfast bowl with Greek yogurt, fresh berries, and a sprinkle of nuts provides a satisfying and nutritious start to your day.

In addition to understanding the importance of each macronutrient, it's essential to listen to your body and pay attention to how different foods make you feel. Everyone's needs are unique, and finding the right balance may require some trial and error. Keep a food journal to track how various meals impact your energy levels, mood, and overall well-being. This process of self-discovery can provide valuable insights as you tailor your eating habits to support your individual goals.

As you move forward, embrace the journey of learning about macronutrients and their role in your health. With knowledge comes power, and understanding how to fuel your body effectively will set you on a path toward success. By prioritizing protein, selecting healthy fats, and focusing on whole carbohydrates, you'll not only enhance your weight loss efforts but also foster a sustainable, healthy lifestyle. Each meal becomes an opportunity to nourish yourself, and as you do, you'll find that success is not just a destination but an ongoing journey of growth and discovery.

Effective Exercise Routines to Boost Metabolism on the Atkins Diet

Regular physical activity is crucial for overall health and weight management, especially when following the Atkins Diet. Exercise helps boost metabolism, increases energy levels, and enhances weight loss. A well-rounded fitness routine should include cardiovascular exercise, strength training, and flexibility exercises.

CARDIOVASCULAR EXERCISE

Activities like brisk walking, jogging, cycling, and swimming are excellent for improving cardiovascular health and burning calories. Target 30 minutes of moderate exercise per session, ideally three to four times weekly.

Brisk Walking: Walk uphill, use stairs, or walk on a treadmill to increase intensity.

Jogging or Running: Start with shorter intervals and gradually increase duration.

Cycling: Stationary bike or outdoor cycling, adjust resistance for challenge.

Swimming: Focus on laps or water aerobics for added intensity.

STRENGTH TRAINING

Building muscle mass through strength training helps increase metabolism and burn fat. Focus on exercises that work multiple muscle groups simultaneously.

Squats: Works legs, glutes, and core muscles.

Lunges: Targets legs, glutes, and hips.

Push-ups: Engages chest, shoulders, and triceps.

Chest Press: Uses dumbbells or resistance bands.

Rows: Works back and arm muscles.

FLEXIBILITY AND STRETCHING EXERCISES

Regular stretching improves flexibility, reduces muscle soreness, and enhances overall mobility.

Yoga integrates flexibility, strength-building postures, and calming techniques for overall wellness.

Pilates: Focuses on core strength, flexibility, and body control.

Dynamic Stretching encompasses movements like leg swings, arm circles, and hip rotations to loosen muscles.

HIGH-INTENSITY INTERVAL TRAINING (HIIT)

HIIT is all about short, intense workouts followed by quick breaks. This type of training boosts metabolism, improves cardiovascular health, and increases caloric burn.

Sprints: Short bursts of running or cycling.

Burpees: Full-body exercise combining strength and cardio.

Jump Squats: Explosive leg exercise.

LOW-IMPACT EXERCISES FOR SENIORS

Gentle exercises tailored to seniors' needs help maintain mobility, balance, and strength.

Water Aerobics: Low-impact, joint-friendly exercise.

Chair Yoga: Modified yoga poses for flexibility and balance.

Resistance Band Exercises: Lightweight, portable, and easy to use.

SAMPLE WORKOUT ROUTINE

Monday (Cardio Day): Brisk walking or jogging (30 minutes)

Tuesday (Strength Training): Squats, lunges, push-ups, chest press (3 sets of 10 reps)

Wednesday (Rest Day)

Thursday (Flexibility): Yoga or Pilates (30 minutes)

Friday (Cardio Day): Swimming or cycling (30 minutes)

Saturday (Strength Training): Rows, leg press, shoulder press (3 sets of 10 reps)

Sunday (Rest Day)

Remember to consult a healthcare professional before starting any new exercise program, especially if you have health concerns or chronic conditions. Listen to your body, adjust intensity and frequency as needed, and stay hydrated throughout your fitness journey.

Regular exercise and a balanced Atkins Diet will help boost your metabolism, enhance weight loss, and improve overall well-being. Stay committed, track progress, and celebrate small victories along the way.

Stocking Your Low-Carb Pantry and Meal Planning

When embarking on a low-carb journey, one of the most empowering steps you can take is to set up a well-stocked pantry. Having the right ingredients at your fingertips can simplify meal preparation, make healthy choices easier, and reduce the temptation to reach for unhealthy options. The goal is to create a space that encourages creativity and exploration while supporting your dietary choices.

Begin by clearing out any items that don't align with your low-carb goals. This doesn't mean you have to throw everything away; instead, consider donating foods that others might enjoy. This helps create a clean slate, allowing you to fill your pantry with wholesome ingredients that fit your new lifestyle. Take a moment to assess what's left and visualize what you want to include moving forward.

Now, let's dive into essential items to include in your low-carb pantry. Start with proteins. Stocking up on canned or packaged options like tuna, salmon, and chicken can make quick meals a breeze. Fresh meats, poultry, and eggs should be staples in your fridge. Don't forget about plant-based protein sources like tofu and tempeh, which can add variety to your meals. Incorporating a mix of these proteins ensures you have plenty of options for different meals throughout the week.

Next, focus on healthy fats. Oils such as olive oil, coconut oil, and avocado oil are fantastic for cooking and dressings. Nuts and seeds, like almonds, walnuts, chia seeds, and flaxseeds, can be excellent snacks or toppings for salads and yogurt. Nut butters also make a delicious addition, providing healthy fat and flavor without unnecessary sugars. Including avocados is a great way to add creaminess and a wealth of nutrients to various dishes.

Spices and herbs are often overlooked but can significantly enhance the flavors of your meals. Stock your pantry with a variety of seasonings to elevate the taste of your dishes. Garlic powder, onion powder, paprika, cumin, and Italian herbs can turn a simple meal into something special. Fresh herbs like basil, cilantro, and parsley can also add vibrant flavors to salads and main courses.

When it comes to carbohydrates, focus on those that are low in net carbs. Consider stocking up on vegetables, especially leafy greens like spinach, kale, and arugula. Cruciferous vegetables such as broccoli, cauliflower, and Brussels sprouts are also fantastic choices, providing essential nutrients and fiber while being low in carbohydrates. You can freeze these vegetables to have a ready supply on hand, making meal prep even easier.

Low-carb grains and alternatives can also play a role in your meal planning. Look for products made from almond flour, coconut flour, and cauliflower rice. These can be used in a variety of recipes, from baking to creating mock rice dishes. They can help satisfy cravings for traditional carbohydrate-rich foods while keeping your meals aligned with your goals.

As you build your pantry, consider meal planning as a key component of your success. Dedicate some time each week to outline your meals, focusing on the ingredients you already have and what you need to buy. Planning ahead allows you to make intentional choices rather than impulsive ones when hunger strikes. With a meal plan in place, you'll find it easier to stick to your low-carb lifestyle.

Start by choosing a few recipes that excite you and align with your dietary goals. Aim for a variety of dishes to keep things interesting. Consider breakfast options such as egg muffins or smoothies packed with greens and protein. For lunch, salads topped with grilled chicken or tuna can be both satisfying and nutritious. Dinner might include stir-fries loaded with vegetables and your choice of protein or hearty soups that warm you up and fill you up.

Don't forget to account for snacks. Healthy options like cheese sticks, nuts, hard-boiled eggs, or veggies with dip can keep you satisfied between meals. Preparing snacks in advance can help you avoid reaching for convenience foods that don't align with your goals. Portioning snacks into grab-and-go containers makes it easy to stay on track.

Finally, keep your pantry organized. Arranging items by category can save you time when you're in a rush to prepare meals. Labeling containers and jars can also help you quickly locate what you need. An organized pantry not only looks inviting but also fosters a sense of control over your food choices.

Setting up a low-carb pantry and planning your meals can significantly enhance your journey. With the right ingredients on hand and a thoughtful approach to meal planning, you're setting yourself up for success. Embrace the process, experiment with new recipes, and enjoy the satisfaction of nourishing your body with wholesome, delicious foods. Each meal becomes an opportunity to savor flavors and celebrate your commitment to a healthier lifestyle, making your journey not just effective but enjoyable.

Breaking Up with Sugar and Processed Foods

Embarking on a journey towards a healthier lifestyle often involves a significant shift in your relationship with food, particularly when it comes to sugar and processed foods. These ingredients, often hidden in plain sight, can be challenging to let go of, but breaking free from their grip is essential for achieving your wellness goals. The good news is that with the right strategies and mindset, you can navigate this transition smoothly and emerge empowered.

Sugar has a way of sneaking into our diets, often disguised under various names in ingredient lists. While it may provide a quick energy boost, the reality is that sugar can lead to energy crashes, increased cravings, and mood swings. When consumed in excess, it can contribute to weight gain and various health issues, including diabetes and heart disease. Recognizing the effects of sugar on your body is the first step in making a change.

Start by examining your current diet and identifying sources of added sugars. Common culprits include sugary drinks, snacks, desserts, and even seemingly healthy options like granola bars and flavored yogurts. Once you become aware of where sugar lurks, you can make conscious decisions to reduce or eliminate those items from your pantry. Replace sugary drinks with sparkling water infused with fresh fruit or herbal teas. For snacks, consider opting for whole foods like nuts, seeds, and fresh fruits, which provide natural sweetness along with essential nutrients.

Transitioning away from sugar may not be an overnight process, and that's perfectly okay. Allow yourself to gradually decrease your intake. Instead of cutting sugar out entirely at once, try to reduce it slowly. This strategy streamlines the process eliminating unnecessary complexity. Over time, your palate will adjust, and you may find that you no longer crave the same levels of sweetness you once did.

Another key player in your diet is processed foods, which often contain not only added sugars but also unhealthy fats, preservatives, and artificial ingredients. These foods can be enticing due to their convenience, but they rarely offer the nourishment your body truly needs. Breaking up with processed foods means embracing whole, unprocessed options that can fuel your body and support your goals.

To start this transformation, focus on cooking more meals at home. Preparing your own food allows you to control the ingredients, making it easier to avoid added sugars and unhealthy additives. Begin with simple recipes that use fresh, whole ingredients. Experimenting in the kitchen can be both fun and rewarding, and you might discover new favorite meals along the way.

When you do buy packaged foods, make a habit of reading labels carefully. Look for items with short ingredient lists, and prioritize those that contain whole ingredients you recognize. Avoid products with added sugars, high fructose corn syrup, and other artificial sweeteners. Learning to decipher food labels empowers you to make informed choices, and over time, you'll develop a keen eye for spotting the healthiest options.

As you work on breaking free from sugar and processed foods, consider the importance of satisfying your cravings in a healthier way. If you find yourself craving something sweet, reach for fresh fruit or a small piece of dark chocolate instead of sugary desserts. Many fruits provide natural sweetness along with fiber, vitamins, and minerals, making them an excellent alternative to processed sweets.

Additionally, find ways to make your meals and snacks more enjoyable. Explore spices like cinnamon or vanilla to add flavor without added sugar. Creative recipes using wholesome ingredients can provide the satisfaction you seek while steering clear of the pitfalls of refined sugar. For instance, baking with almond flour or coconut flour can create delicious treats without the sugar overload.

Support from friends and family can also make a significant difference during this transition. Share your goals with those close to you, and invite them to join you in this healthier lifestyle. Cooking together, sharing recipes, and encouraging each other can foster a sense of camaraderie that makes breaking up with sugar and processed foods more enjoyable.

Mindfulness is another powerful tool in this journey. Take time to savor each bite and recognize the flavors and textures of your food. Mindful eating can help you appreciate the natural sweetness of whole foods and make you more aware of how certain foods affect your body. This practice not only enhances your meals but also strengthens your relationship with food.

Finally, don't forget to be kind to yourself during this process. Change takes time, and it's normal to have moments of temptation or craving. Acknowledge those feelings without judgment and remember that every step you take toward reducing sugar and processed foods is a step in the right direction. Celebrate your successes, no matter how small, and keep your focus on the positive changes you're making for your health.

Breaking up with sugar and processed foods may initially feel daunting, but with determination, creativity, and support, you can navigate this journey successfully. Embrace the opportunity to discover new flavors, enhance your culinary skills, and nourish your body with wholesome ingredients. As you let go of the unhealthy habits, you'll find that your energy levels improve, your cravings diminish, and your overall well-being flourishes, paving the way for a healthier, happier you.

Chapter 3: The New Atkins Diet Phases

Phase 1: Induction - Jumpstarting Your Weight Loss

You're ready to ignite your weight loss journey. Phase 1, Induction, is the launchpad for transformative change. This critical phase sets the stage for a healthier, leaner you.

Induction is a 14-day kickstart, designed to:

- Reset your metabolism
- Stabilize blood sugar
- Unlock fat burning
- Boost energy
- Enhance mental clarity

The rules are simple:

- Eat protein-rich foods

- Focus on healthy fats
- Incorporate vegetables
- Eliminate added sugars
- Limit carbohydrate intake

Entering the first phase of your journey toward healthier living can feel exhilarating yet challenging. This initial stage emphasizes a significant reduction in carbohydrate intake, allowing your body to shift into a state of ketosis, where it begins to burn fat for energy instead of carbohydrates. Understanding this phase can empower you to embrace the changes and seize the opportunity for success.

During the Induction phase, the focus is on drastically reducing your daily carbohydrate intake to around twenty grams per day, primarily from leafy green vegetables. This initial restriction prompts your body to transition from burning glucose to utilizing stored fat as its primary energy source. As this metabolic shift occurs, you may experience weight loss within the first week, which can be both motivating and invigorating. Many people notice a drop on the scale almost immediately, which serves as a powerful incentive to continue on the journey.

One of the key aspects of the Induction phase is the emphasis on consuming nutrient-dense foods. Prioritizing high-quality proteins and healthy fats is essential for supporting your body during this transition. Foods such as lean meats, fish, eggs, avocados, nuts, and seeds should take center stage on your plate. These options not only provide essential nutrients but also promote feelings of fullness, helping to curb cravings and prevent hunger.

It's important to recognize that while the Induction phase may feel restrictive at first, it's designed to reset your palate and help you become accustomed to lower-carb foods. As you eliminate processed carbohydrates and sugars, you may find that your taste buds begin to adjust, making whole foods more appealing. This process can lead to a newfound appreciation for the flavors and textures of fresh ingredients.

To ensure you have a variety of meals during this phase, explore different cooking methods and recipes. Grilling, roasting, or sautéing vegetables with olive oil can bring out their natural flavors, while herbs and spices can elevate your dishes without adding extra carbs. Consider creating simple, satisfying meals that include a protein source paired with non-starchy vegetables. For instance, a grilled chicken breast served with sautéed spinach and garlic makes for a nutritious and delicious meal.

As you embark on the Induction phase, staying hydrated is crucial. Drinking plenty of water not only supports overall health but also helps mitigate any initial side effects that may arise as your body adjusts to a lower carb intake. Some individuals experience symptoms like headaches or fatigue, commonly referred to as the "keto flu." Staying well-hydrated can alleviate some of these discomforts and keep your energy levels stable.

Monitoring your progress during this phase can also be beneficial. Consider keeping a journal to track your meals, energy levels, and feelings throughout the process. Not only does this practice help maintain accountability, but it also allows you to identify patterns and discover which foods make you feel your best. Celebrate your successes, no matter how small, as they can serve as motivation to push forward.

Additionally, while this phase encourages a reduction in carbohydrates, it does not mean you should shy away from enjoying your meals. Find ways to make the process enjoyable by experimenting with different recipes and flavors. Explore new cuisines that emphasize low-carb ingredients, such as Mediterranean or Asian dishes. Engaging your creativity in the kitchen can turn meal prep into a delightful experience rather than a chore.

Social situations may present challenges during the Induction phase, especially if you're accustomed to certain dining habits. Talking openly with friends and family about your dietary choices can create a stronger support system. Consider suggesting low-carb-friendly restaurants or planning meals that cater to your new lifestyle. Embracing this phase doesn't mean isolating yourself; it's about finding balance and adapting to your surroundings while staying true to your goals.

Lastly, remember that this phase is just the beginning of your journey. The Induction phase is designed to set a strong foundation for your future success. As you progress, you'll gain insights into your body's response to different foods, which will help you make informed choices in the next phases. Approach this journey with an open mind and a willingness to learn; every experience is a valuable lesson that contributes to your overall growth.

The Induction phase serves as a powerful catalyst for change. By committing to this phase and embracing its principles, you're taking a proactive step toward transforming your relationship with food and your body. Celebrate the small victories, stay focused on your goals, and remember that you have the power to reshape your future. As you navigate this initial phase, you'll find yourself not only jumpstarting your weight loss but also embarking on a journey toward lasting health and vitality.

Phase 2: Balancing – Finding Your Carb Tolerance

You've conquered Induction and are now ready to enter the Balancing phase. This critical stage helps you find your carb tolerance, ensuring a sustainable, long-term weight loss journey.

In Balancing, you'll:

- Gradually increase carbohydrate intake
- Introduce new foods
- Refine your eating habits
- Monitor progress

The goal is to find your individual carb tolerance, the point at which your body can handle carbohydrates without hindering weight loss or overall health.

To begin, reassess your food list:

- Add nutrient-dense carbohydrates
- Include healthy grains
- Explore fruit and vegetable options

Focus on whole, unprocessed foods:

- Whole grains (brown rice, quinoa, whole wheat)
- Fruits (apples, berries, citrus)
- Vegetables (leafy greens, broccoli, bell peppers)

Your Balancing shopping list should include

Proteins:

- Chicken breast
- Lean beef (grass-fed)
- Fish (salmon, tilapia)
- Eggs
- Turkey sausage
- Bacon
- Tofu
- Shrimp
- Pork tenderloin
- Chicken thighs
- Ground turkey
- Steak (ribeye, sirloin)
- Lamb chops
- Venison
- Turkey bacon
- Chicken drumsticks
- Pork chops
- Beef strips (sirloin)
- Fish sticks (low-carb)
- Lobster

Vegetables:

- Leafy greens (spinach, kale)
- Broccoli
- Bell peppers
- Cucumbers
- Tomatoes
- Avocados
- Mushrooms
- Asparagus
- Zucchini
- Green beans
- Carrots
- Celery
- Radishes
- Cabbage
- Bok choy
- Cauliflower
- Brussels sprouts
- Sweet potatoes
- Turnips
- Watercress

Fruits:

- Berries (strawberries, blueberries) ✓
- Citrus fruits (oranges, grapefruits)

- Apples ✔
- Pears ✔
- Peaches ✔
- Apricots ✔
- Plums
- Cherries
- Acai berries ✔
- Cranberries
- Raspberries ✔
- Blackberries ✔
- Lemons
- Limes
- Avocado ✔
- Papaya
- Mango
- Pineapple
- Watermelon
- Cantaloupe

Grains:

- Almond flour
- Coconut flour
- Cauliflower rice
- Zucchini noodles
- Spaghetti squash
- Shirataki noodles

Keto

- Low-carb tortillas ✔
- Low-carb bread ✔
- Coconut flakes
- Chia seed crackers
- Flaxseed crackers
- Low-carb cereal
- Protein pasta
- Vegetable wraps
- Portobello mushroom caps
- Low-carb pizza crust
- Cauliflower pizza crust
- Zucchini bread ✔
- Coconut macaroons
- Low-carb granola

Dairy/ Alternative:

- Almond milk
- Greek yogurt
- Cottage cheese
- Full-fat cheese (cheddar, mozzarella)
- Coconut milk
- Cream cheese
- Ricotta cheese
- Feta cheese
- Goat cheese
- Protein powder (whey, casein)

- Coconut yogurt
- Cashew milk
- Oat milk
- Macadamia nut milk
- Vegan cheese
- Kefir
- Butter
- Cream
- Sour cream
- Half-and-half

Healthy Fats:

- Olive oil ✔
- Coconut oil ✔
- Avocado oil ✔
- Nuts (almonds, walnuts) ✔
- Seeds (chia, flax)
- Fatty fish (salmon, tuna) ✔
- Full-fat dairy ✔
- Bacon fat
- ~~Duck fat~~
- ~~Ghee~~
- Lard
- Macadamia nuts
- Pecans
- Hazelnuts

- Pistachios
- Sunflower seeds
- Pumpkin seeds
- Chia seed oil
- Flaxseed oil
- Walnut oil

Condiments:
- Salt
- Pepper
- Garlic powder
- Onion powder
- Herbs (basil, oregano)
- Lemon juice
- Lime juice
- Vinegar (apple cider, balsamic)
- Hot sauce
- Soy sauce
- Tomato sauce
- Salsa
- Guacamole
- Hummus
- Mayonnaise
- Mustard
- Relish
- Pickles
- Olives
- Capers

Snacks:

- Raw veggies with hummus
- Cheese sticks
- Hard-boiled eggs
- Handful of nuts
- Protein bars (Atkins-approved)
- Jerky (beef, turkey)
- Low-carb crackers
- Cheese puffs
- Pork rinds
- Low-carb chips
- Popcorn (air-popped)
- Trail mix
- Mozzarella cheese balls
- Atkins Diet shakes
- Low-carb granola bars
- Cottage cheese cups
- Fresh berries with cream cheese
- Celery sticks with almond butter
- Protein smoothie packs
- Zucchini chips

Pantry:

- Almond flour
- Coconut flour
- Low-carb crackers

- Canned black beans
- Canned tomatoes

Sample meals:

Avocado and Bacon Omelet

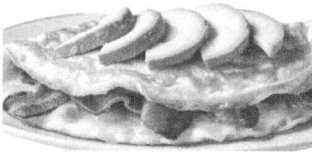

Ingredients:
- 2 eggs
- 1/2 avocado, sliced
- 4 slices of bacon
- Salt and pepper to taste

Preparation:
In a bowl, whisk eggs and season with salt and pepper.
Heat a non-stick pan with coconut oil over medium heat.
Add bacon and cook until crispy.
Pour in eggs and cook until set.
Fold omelet in half and top with avocado slices.

Greek Yogurt Parfait

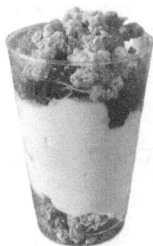

Ingredients:
- 1 cup Greek yogurt
- 1/2 cup mixed berries
- 1/4 cup chopped almonds
- 1 tablespoon honey

Preparation:
Layer yogurt, berries, and almonds in a bowl.
Drizzle with honey.

Whole-Grain Toast with Avocado and Poached Eggs

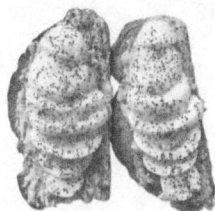

Ingredients:
- 2 slices whole-grain bread
- 1 avocado, mashed
- 2 eggs
- Salt and pepper to taste

Preparation:
Toast bread and top with mashed avocado.
Poach eggs and place on top.
Season with salt and pepper

LUNCH OPTIONS:

Creamy Garlic Mushroom Chicken

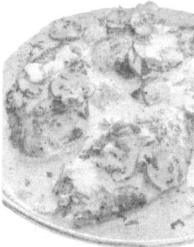

Ingredients:
- 4 boneless, skinless chicken thighs
- 2 tbsp olive oil
- 1 cup mushrooms, sliced
- 3 cloves garlic, minced
- 1 cup heavy cream
- 1/2 cup grated Parmesan cheese
- 1 tsp dried thyme or rosemary
- Salt and pepper to taste

Preparation:
Heat olive oil in a large skillet over medium-high heat. Season chicken thighs with salt and pepper, and cook until golden brown and cooked through (about 5-7 minutes per side). Remove from the skillet and set aside.

Add sliced mushrooms to the same skillet; cook until tender (5 min). Then add minced garlic (1 min).

Reduce heat to medium, pour in the heavy cream, and stir to combine. Add Parmesan cheese and thyme or rosemary. Simmer until the sauce thickens slightly.

Put the chicken thighs back in the skillet and coat with sauce. Simmer for a few minutes to heat through and blend flavors.

Turkey and Avocado Wrap

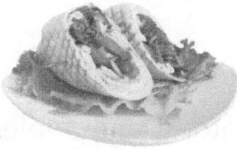

Ingredients:
- 1 whole-grain tortilla

- 2 oz sliced turkey breast
- 1/2 avocado, sliced
- 1 cup mixed greens
- 1/4 cup sliced red onion

Preparation:
Assemble wrap with turkey, avocado, greens, and onion.

Salmon Salad with Mixed Greens and Whole-Grain Crackers

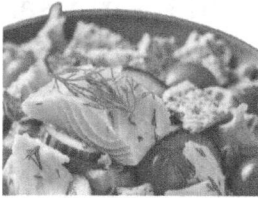

Ingredients:
- 4 oz cooked salmon
- 2 cups mixed greens
- 1/4 cup cherry tomatoes
- 1/4 cup diced apple
- 2 whole-grain crackers

Preparation:
Mix salmon, greens, cherry tomatoes, and apples in a bowl.
Serve with whole-grain crackers.

Grilled Chicken Breast with Roasted Broccoli and Quinoa

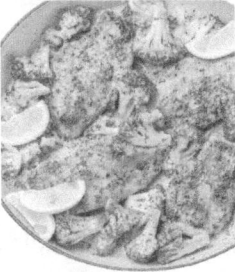

Ingredients:
- 4 oz grilled chicken breast
- 1 cup quinoa
- 1 cup broccoli florets
- 2 tablespoons olive oil
- Salt and pepper to taste

Preparation:
Grill chicken breast and slice.
Cook quinoa according to package instructions.
Roast broccoli in olive oil and season with salt and pepper.

Beef and Vegetable Stir-Fry

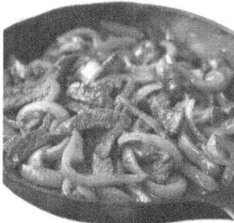

Ingredients:
- 4 oz beef strips
- 1 cup mixed vegetables (bell peppers, carrots, snow peas)
- 2 tablespoons coconut oil
- 1 tablespoon soy sauce
- 1 teaspoon garlic powder

Preparation:
Heat coconut oil in a wok or large skillet.
Cook beef strips until browned.
Add mixed vegetables and cook until tender.
Season with soy sauce and garlic powder.

Baked Chicken Thighs with Roasted Carrots and Brussels Sprouts

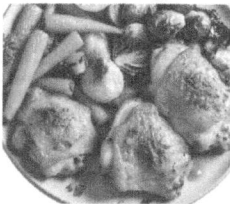

Ingredients:
- 4 oz baked chicken thighs
- 1 cup carrots, peeled and chopped
- 1 cup Brussels sprouts, halved
- 2 tablespoons olive oil
- Salt and pepper to taste

Preparation:
Bake chicken thighs in the oven with olive oil and season with salt and pepper.
Roast carrots and Brussels sprouts in olive oil.

Shrimp and Vegetable Skewers

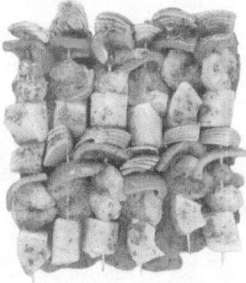

Ingredients:
- 4 oz shrimp, peeled and deveined
- 1 cup mixed vegetables (zucchini, bell peppers, onions)
- 2 tablespoons olive oil
- 1 tablespoon lemon juice
- Salt and pepper to taste

Preparation:
Alternate shrimp and vegetables on skewers.
Brush with olive oil and season with lemon juice.
Grill or bake until cooked through.

Turkey Meatballs with Zucchini Noodles

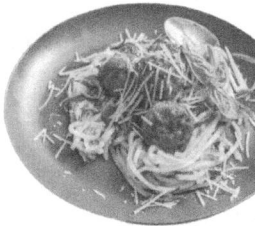

Ingredients:
- 4 oz turkey meatballs
- 1 cup zucchini noodles
- 2 tablespoons olive oil
- 1 cup marinara sauce
- 1/4 cup grated Parmesan cheese

Preparation:
Cook turkey meatballs in olive oil.
Sauté zucchini noodles in olive oil.
Serve meatballs with zucchini noodles and marinara sauce.

Apple Slices with Almond Butter

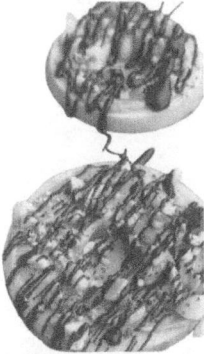

Ingredients:
- 1 apple, sliced
- 2 tablespoons almond butter
- chocolate (optional)

Preparation:
Spread almond butter on apple slices.

Greek Yogurt with Berries

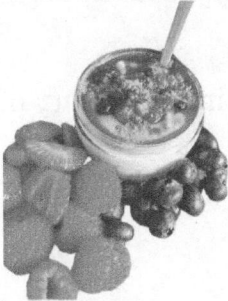

Ingredients:
- 1 cup Greek yogurt

- 1/2 cup mixed berries

Preparation:
- Mix yogurt and berries.

Hard-Boiled Eggs

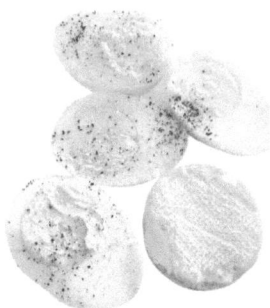

Ingredients:
- 2 eggs

Preparation:
Boil eggs and slice. Season with pepper (optional)

Remember to stay hydrated by drinking plenty of water throughout the day.

Tips for success:

- Keep a food diary
- Track carb intake

- Stay hydrated
- Exercise regularly

By finding your carb tolerance, you'll:

- Unlock personalized weight loss
- Improve blood sugar control
- Enhance metabolic flexibility

You're one step closer to maintaining a healthy, balanced lifestyle.

NB: **You mustn't buy everything on the list if you're trying to fit into a specific budget, you can pick out your choices from each section**.

Phase 3: Fine-Tuning – Maintaining Your Weight Loss

Reaching your weight loss goals is a significant achievement, but maintaining that success requires a thoughtful approach. As you enter this phase, the focus shifts from strict adherence to new habits to fine-tuning your lifestyle for lasting results. This journey is about finding balance and sustainability while still enjoying the foods you love.

Start by listening to your body. Understand what it needs, both physically and emotionally. As you transition into maintenance, pay attention to hunger cues and satisfaction levels. Learning to distinguish between true hunger and emotional eating can make all the difference. Mindful eating becomes essential. By savoring each bite and being present during meals, you not only enhance your enjoyment of food but also prevent overeating.

Experiment with your meal plans. This is the time to explore and discover which foods work best for you. You might find that certain low-carb options make you feel more energized and satisfied than others. Keep track of how different meals affect your mood and energy levels. This process will help you create a personalized approach that aligns with your lifestyle and preferences.

Physical activity plays a pivotal role in maintenance. Find exercises that you genuinely enjoy, whether it's dancing, hiking, or yoga. When movement becomes a source of joy rather than a chore, it's easier to stay consistent. Aim to make activity a regular part of your routine, not just for weight maintenance but also for overall well-being.

Building a support network can also enhance your success. Build a supportive network by connecting with like-minded individuals, loved ones, or online groups who share your objectives. Sharing experiences, challenges, and triumphs can motivate you to stay on track. Remember, it's perfectly normal to experience fluctuations along the way. Instead of dwelling on setbacks, reframe them as valuable lessons that help refine your strategy.

Finally, celebrate your progress. Recognize that maintaining weight loss is a journey filled with ups and downs. Reward yourself for small milestones, not just the big ones. Embrace this phase with confidence, knowing you have the tools to sustain your achievements and continue thriving in your healthier lifestyle.

Phase 4: Maintenance – Living the Low-Carb Lifestyle

As you transition into the maintenance phase, the goal is to embrace a lifestyle that supports your health and well-being while enjoying the benefits of your hard-earned weight loss. This stage is not about rigid rules but about fostering habits that fit seamlessly into your life. The key to long-term success lies in adopting a low-carb lifestyle that feels natural and sustainable.

Begin by celebrating your achievements. Recognizing the hard work you've put in can motivate you to stay committed. Reflect on the changes you've made and how they've positively impacted your life. This is your moment to take pride in your accomplishments while looking forward to a fulfilling journey ahead.

Adapting to a low-carb lifestyle doesn't mean deprivation. It's about discovering a variety of delicious and satisfying foods that align with your preferences. Explore new recipes and ingredients that excite your palate. From vibrant salads to flavorful meats and hearty vegetables, there's a wealth of options that can keep your meals enjoyable. Learning to cook with fresh herbs and spices can enhance flavors without adding extra carbs. Experimenting in the kitchen can also become a fun activity, making mealtime an adventure rather than a routine.

Consistency is crucial, but it's equally important to remain flexible. Life is full of social events and gatherings, and you don't want to feel isolated by strict dietary rules. Instead, approach these situations with a mindset of balance. Choose low-carb options when available, but don't hesitate to indulge occasionally. It's about finding that sweet spot where you can enjoy treats without derailing your progress. Learning to navigate dining out or special occasions with confidence will help reinforce your commitment to this lifestyle.

Physical activity should continue to be a priority in your daily routine. Find ways to embed movement into your day that you genuinely enjoy. Whether it's walking, cycling, or engaging in a fun fitness class, staying active will not only help you maintain your weight but also enhance your overall health. Setting new fitness goals can be a motivating factor as you explore different activities and push your limits.

As you navigate this phase, remember that the journey is not always linear. You might encounter moments where the scale fluctuates or you feel tempted to revert to old habits. This is completely normal and part of the process. When faced with challenges, remind yourself of the tools and knowledge you've gained. Instead of viewing these moments as setbacks, consider them opportunities for growth. Reassess your goals, make adjustments, and continue moving forward with a positive mindset.

Additionally, maintaining a supportive environment is essential. Surround yourself with individuals who understand and encourage your lifestyle choices. Whether it's family, friends, or online communities, having a support system can help you stay accountable and motivated. Sharing experiences and exchanging tips can foster a sense of camaraderie that reinforces your commitment.

Finally, prioritize self-care. This journey is about more than just food; it encompasses your overall well-being. Engage in activities that promote mental and emotional health, such as mindfulness practices, journaling, or spending time in nature. These practices can enhance your resilience and help you navigate challenges with grace.

Living the low-carb lifestyle in maintenance is a celebration of your achievements and a commitment to your health. By focusing on enjoyment, flexibility, and a supportive community, you can create a fulfilling life that allows you to thrive long after reaching your weight loss goals. Embrace this phase as an opportunity to continue learning and growing, knowing that the best is yet to come.

Chapter 4: Meal Planning and Recipes

Breakfast Ideas: Delicious Low-Carb Options

These low carb ideas will keep your mornings flavorful and satisfying while aligning with your lifestyle.

Spinach and Feta Omelette

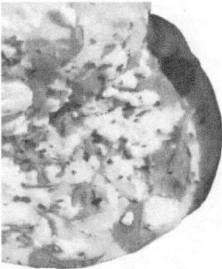

Ingredients:
- 2 large eggs
- 1 cup fresh spinach, chopped
- 1/4 cup feta cheese, crumbled
- Salt and pepper to taste
- 1 tablespoon olive oil

Preparation:

Heat olive oil in a non-stick skillet over medium heat.

Whisk eggs in a bowl and season with salt and pepper.

Pour eggs into the skillet, swirling to coat.

Add spinach and feta on one half of the omelet.

Cook until eggs are set, about 3-4 minutes. Fold and serve.

Avocado and Egg Breakfast Bowl

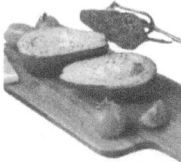

Ingredients:

- 1 ripe avocado, halved and pitted
- 2 eggs
- Salt and pepper to taste
- Red pepper flakes (optional)

Preparation:

Boil water in a small pot. Carefully add eggs and boil for 6-7 minutes for soft-boiling.

While eggs are cooking, scoop out some avocado flesh to create a bowl.

Once eggs are done, peel and slice them.

Place egg slices into avocado halves, season with salt, pepper, and red pepper flakes if desired.

Chia Seed Pudding

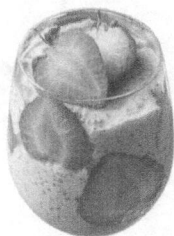

Ingredients:
- 1/4 cup chia seeds
- 1 cup unsweetened almond milk
- 1/2 teaspoon vanilla extract
- A few berries for topping

Preparation:

In a bowl, mix chia seeds, almond milk, and vanilla extract.

Stir well and refrigerate for at least 4 hours or overnight.

Top with berries before serving.

Sausage and Veggie Scramble

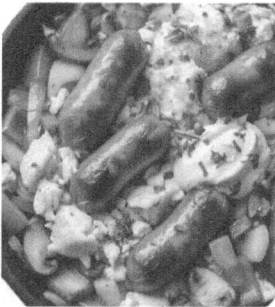

Ingredients:

- 2 sausage links, sliced
- 1/2 bell pepper, chopped
- 1/2 onion, chopped
- 2 large eggs
- Salt and pepper to taste

Preparation:

In a skillet, cook sausage over medium heat until browned.

Add bell pepper and onion; sauté until soft.

Whisk eggs in a bowl, pour into the skillet, and scramble until cooked through.

Season with salt and pepper.

Greek Yogurt Parfait

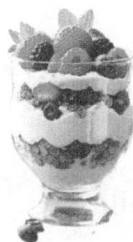

Ingredients:

- 1 cup full-fat Greek yogurt
- 1/4 cup mixed nuts (almonds, walnuts, etc.)
- 1/4 cup berries (strawberries, blueberries)

Preparation:

In a glass, layer Greek yogurt, nuts, and berries.

Repeat layers and enjoy immediately.

Almond Flour Pancakes

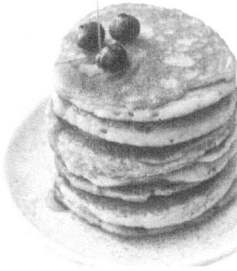

Ingredients:
- 1 cup almond flour
- 2 eggs
- 1/4 cup unsweetened almond milk
- 1 teaspoon baking powder
- Butter for cooking

Preparation:
In a bowl, mix almond flour, eggs, almond milk, and baking powder until smooth.
Heat a skillet over medium heat and add butter.

Pour batter into the skillet, cooking until bubbles form, then flip and cook until golden.

Serve with sugar-free syrup or berries.

Zucchini Fritters

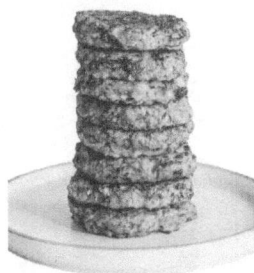

Ingredients:
- 1 medium zucchini, grated
- 1 egg
- 1/4 cup almond flour
- 1/4 cup cheese (cheddar or mozzarella)
- Salt and pepper to taste

Preparation:
Squeeze excess moisture from grated zucchini.

In a bowl, combine zucchini, egg, almond flour, cheese, salt, and pepper.

Heat oil in a skillet and spoon mixture into the pan.

Cook until golden brown on both sides, about 3-4 minutes per side.

Cottage Cheese Bowl

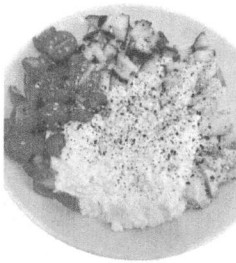

Ingredients:

- 1 cup cottage cheese
- 1/4 cup sliced cucumber
- 1/4 cup cherry tomatoes, halved
- Olive oil, salt, and pepper

Preparation:

In a bowl, add cottage cheese and top with cucumber and tomatoes.

Drizzle with olive oil and season with salt and pepper.

Smoked Salmon and Cream Cheese Wrap

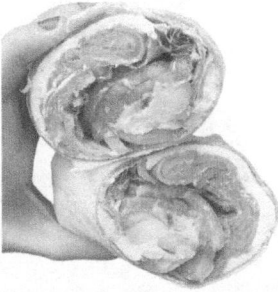

Ingredients:

- 1 low-carb tortilla
- 2 ounces smoked salmon
- 2 tablespoons cream cheese
- A handful of arugula

Preparation:

Spread cream cheese on the tortilla.

Layer smoked salmon and arugula on top.

Roll tightly and slice in half.

Cauliflower Hash Browns

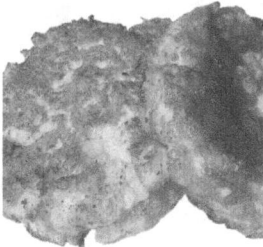

Ingredients:
- 1 cup cauliflower rice
- 1 egg
- 1/4 cup cheese (optional)
- Salt and pepper to taste

Preparation:

Preheat the oven to 400°F (200°C).

In a bowl, combine cauliflower rice, egg, cheese, salt, and pepper.

Form into patties and place on a baking sheet.

Bake for 20 minutes, flipping halfway through until golden brown.

Peanut Butter Smoothie

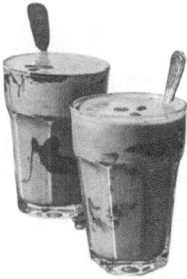

Ingredients:
- 1 cup unsweetened almond milk
- 2 tablespoons natural peanut butter
- 1 tablespoon cocoa powder
- Ice cubes

Preparation:
In a blender, combine almond milk, peanut butter, cocoa powder, and ice.
Blend until smooth and creamy.

Egg Muffins

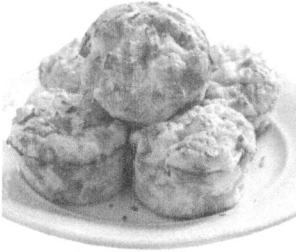

Ingredients:

- 6 large eggs
- 1/2 cup diced bell pepper
- 1/2 cup diced onion
- Salt and pepper to taste
- 1/2 cup shredded cheese

Preparation:

Preheat the oven to 350°F (175°C).

In a bowl, whisk eggs and season with salt and pepper.

Stir in bell pepper, onion, and cheese.

Pour mixture into greased muffin tins and bake for 20-25 minutes until golden brown.

Berry Smoothie Bowl

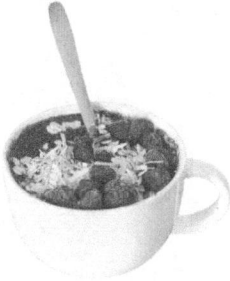

Ingredients:

- 1 cup frozen berries
- 1/2 cup unsweetened almond milk
- Toppings: sliced almonds, shredded coconut, fresh berries

Preparation:

In a blender, combine frozen berries and almond milk.

Blend until thick and creamy.

Pour into a bowl and add toppings of choice.

Breakfast Stuffed Peppers

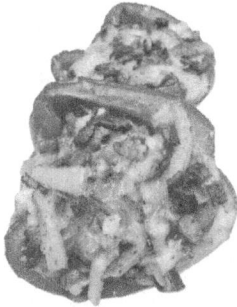

Ingredients:

- 2 bell peppers, halved and seeded
- 4 eggs
- 1/2 cup cooked sausage or bacon
- 1/2 cup shredded cheese

Preparation:

Preheat the oven to 375°F (190°C).

In a bowl, whisk eggs and stir in sausage or bacon and cheese.

Fill each pepper half with the egg mixture.

Place in a baking dish and bake for 25-30 minutes until eggs are set.

Broccoli and Cheese Egg Bake

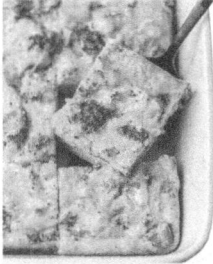

Ingredients:

- 2 cups broccoli florets, steamed
- 6 large eggs
- 1 cup shredded cheese
- Salt and pepper to taste

Preparation:

Preheat the oven to 350°F (175°C).

In a bowl, whisk eggs and season with salt and pepper.

Stir in steamed broccoli and cheese.

Pour mixture into a greased baking dish and bake for 30-35 minutes until set.

These breakfast options not only keep you on track with your low-carb lifestyle but also ensure that your mornings are delicious and enjoyable. With a variety of flavors and textures, you can keep your breakfast routine exciting and satisfying. Enjoy!

Lunch and Dinner Recipes: Easy and Nutritious

Lemon Herb Grilled Chicken

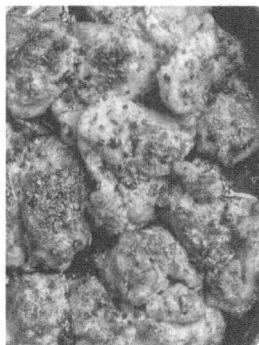

Ingredients:
- 4 boneless chicken breasts
- Juice of 2 lemons
- 2 tablespoons olive oil
- 2 cloves garlic, minced

- 1 tablespoon fresh thyme
- Salt and pepper to taste

Preparation:

In a bowl, mix lemon juice, olive oil, garlic, thyme, salt, and pepper.

Marinate chicken in the mixture for at least 30 minutes.

Preheat the grill to medium-high heat.

Grill chicken for 6-7 minutes per side, until cooked through.

Serve with a side salad.

Cauliflower Fried Rice

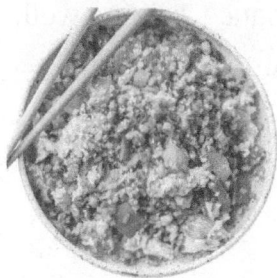

Ingredients:

- 1 head cauliflower, grated into rice-sized pieces

- 2 eggs, beaten
- 1 cup mixed vegetables (peas, carrots, bell peppers)
- 2 tablespoons soy sauce (or tamari for gluten-free)
- 2 tablespoons sesame oil
- Green onions for garnish

Preparation:
Heat sesame oil in a large skillet over medium heat.
Add mixed vegetables and cook until tender.
Push veggies to the side and scramble eggs in the skillet.
Stir in cauliflower rice and soy sauce, mixing well.
Cook for 5-7 minutes until cauliflower is tender.
Garnish with green onions.

Zucchini Noodles with Pesto

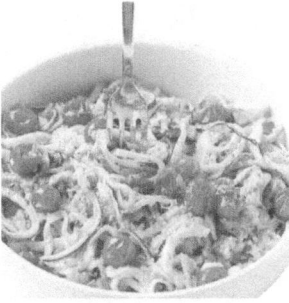

Ingredients:

- 2 medium zucchinis, spiralized
- 1/2 cup pesto
- 1 cup cherry tomatoes, halved
- Grated Parmesan cheese for serving

Preparation:

In a skillet, heat pesto over medium heat.

Add zucchini noodles and cherry tomatoes; cook for 3-4 minutes until tender.

Serve topped with grated Parmesan cheese.

Beef and Broccoli Stir-Fry

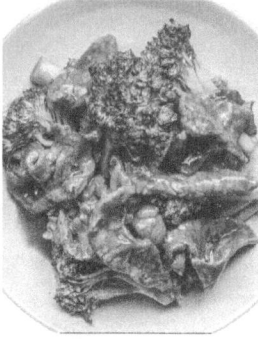

Ingredients:

- 1 pound flank steak, sliced
- 2 cups broccoli florets
- 3 tablespoons soy sauce
- 1 tablespoon ginger, minced
- 2 tablespoons olive oil

Preparation:

Heat olive oil in a large skillet over high heat.

Add beef and cook until browned, about 3-4 minutes.

Add broccoli, ginger, and soy sauce; stir-fry for an additional 5 minutes.

Serve hot.

Caprese Salad with Avocado

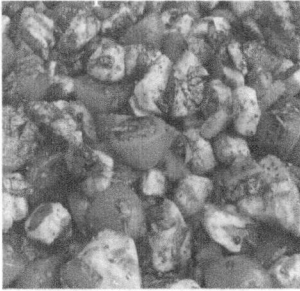

Ingredients:

- 2 large tomatoes, sliced
- 1 ball fresh mozzarella, sliced
- 1 ripe avocado, sliced
- Fresh basil leaves
- Balsamic glaze for drizzling

Preparation:

On a platter, alternate slices of tomato, mozzarella, and avocado.

Top with fresh basil leaves.

Drizzle with balsamic glaze before serving.

Shrimp Tacos in Lettuce Wraps

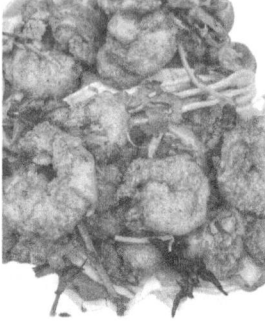

Ingredients:

- 1 pound shrimp, peeled and deveined
- 1 tablespoon olive oil
- 1 teaspoon chili powder
- 1 teaspoon cumin
- Lettuce leaves for wrapping

Preparation:

In a bowl, toss shrimp with olive oil, chili powder, and cumin.

Heat a skillet over medium heat and cook shrimp for 2-3 minutes on each side.

Serve in lettuce leaves with your favorite toppings, such as salsa or avocado.

Eggplant Parmesan

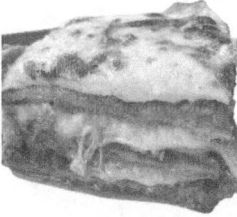

Ingredients:
- 2 medium eggplants, sliced
- 2 cups marinara sauce
- 2 cups shredded mozzarella cheese
- 1/2 cup grated Parmesan cheese
- Olive oil for drizzling

Preparation:
Preheat the oven to 375°F (190°C).

Arrange eggplant slices on a baking sheet, drizzle with olive oil, and bake for 20 minutes.

In a baking dish, layer eggplant, marinara sauce, and cheeses.

Repeat layers, finishing with cheese on top.

Bake for an additional 25 minutes until bubbly and golden.

Stuffed Bell Peppers (cauliflower rice)

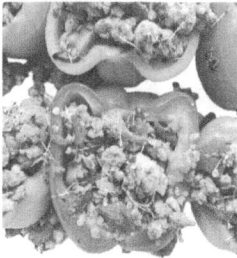

Ingredients:

- 4 bell peppers, halved and seeded
- 1 pound ground turkey or beef
- 1 cup cauliflower rice
- 1 can diced tomatoes
- 1 teaspoon Italian seasoning

Preparation:

Preheat the oven to 375°F (190°C).

In a skillet, brown the ground meat, then add cauliflower rice, tomatoes, and seasoning. Cook until heated through.

Fill bell pepper halves with the mixture and place in a baking dish.

Bake for 25-30 minutes until peppers are tender.

Spinach and Cheese Stuffed Chicken

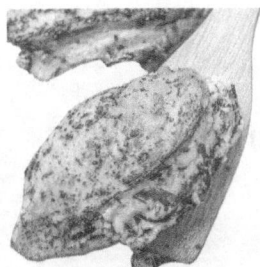

Ingredients:
- 4 boneless chicken breasts
- 1 cup fresh spinach, chopped
- 1/2 cup cream cheese, softened
- 1/2 cup shredded mozzarella cheese
- Salt and pepper to taste

Preparation:

Preheat the oven to 375°F (190°C).

In a bowl, mix spinach, cream cheese, mozzarella, salt, and pepper.

Cut a pocket in each chicken breast and fill with the spinach mixture.

Secure with toothpicks if needed and place in a baking dish.

Bake for 30-35 minutes until chicken is cooked through.

Greek Salad with Grilled Chicken

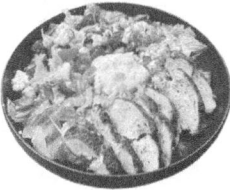

Ingredients:

- 2 cups romaine lettuce, chopped
- 1 cucumber, diced
- 1 cup cherry tomatoes, halved

- 1/2 red onion, sliced
- 1/2 cup Kalamata olives
- 1 pound grilled chicken, sliced
- Olive oil and lemon juice for dressing

Preparation:

In a large bowl, combine lettuce, cucumber, tomatoes, onion, and olives.

Top with grilled chicken slices.

Drizzle with olive oil and lemon juice before serving.

Creamy Tomato Basil Soup

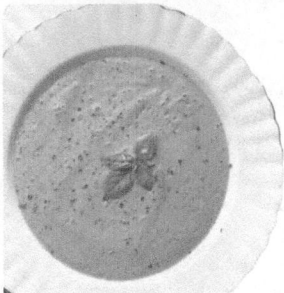

Ingredients:

- 2 cups diced tomatoes (fresh or canned)
- 1 cup vegetable broth

- 1/2 cup heavy cream
- 1/4 cup fresh basil, chopped
- Salt and pepper to taste

Preparation:

In a saucepan, combine tomatoes and vegetable broth; simmer for 15 minutes.

Use an immersion blender to puree until smooth.

Stir in heavy cream and basil, then season with salt and pepper before serving.

Coconut Curry Chicken

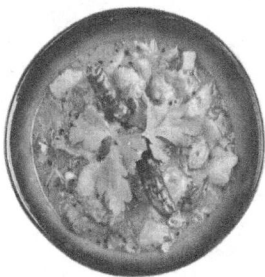

Ingredients:
- 1 pound chicken thighs, cubed
- 1 can coconut milk
- 2 tablespoons curry powder

- 1 cup spinach
- Salt to taste

Preparation:

In a skillet, cook chicken over medium heat until browned.

Stir in coconut milk and curry powder; simmer for 10 minutes.

Add spinach and cook until wilted. Season with salt before serving.

Grilled Salmon with Asparagus

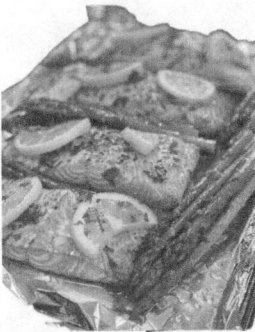

Ingredients:
- 4 salmon filets
- 1 bunch asparagus, trimmed

- 2 tablespoons olive oil
- Salt and pepper to taste

Preparation:
Preheat the grill to medium-high heat.
Toss asparagus with olive oil, salt, and pepper.
Grill salmon for 4-5 minutes per side and asparagus for 2-3 minutes until tender.
Serve together with a lemon wedge.

Chicken Caesar Salad

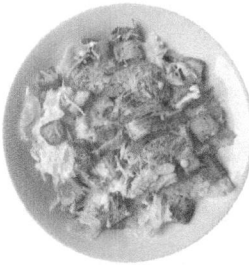

Ingredients:
- 2 cups romaine lettuce, chopped
- 1 cup grilled chicken, sliced
- 1/4 cup Parmesan cheese, grated

- Caesar dressing (low-carb version)

Preparation:

In a bowl, toss lettuce with Caesar dressing until coated.

Top with grilled chicken and sprinkle with Parmesan cheese before serving.

Baked Cod with Lemon and Dill

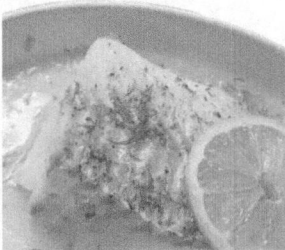

Ingredients:

- 4 cod filets
- Juice of 1 lemon
- 2 tablespoons olive oil
- 2 tablespoons fresh dill, chopped
- Salt and pepper to taste

Preparation:

Preheat the oven to 400°F (200°C).

Place cod filets in a baking dish and drizzle with olive oil and lemon juice.

Sprinkle it with dill, salt, and pepper.

Bake for 12-15 minutes until the fish flakes easily with a fork.

Taco Salad

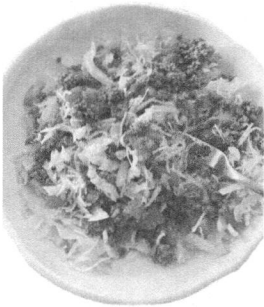

Ingredients:

- 1 pound ground beef or turkey
- 1 packet taco seasoning (low-carb)
- 4 cups romaine lettuce, chopped
- 1 cup diced tomatoes

- 1/2 cup shredded cheese
- 1/4 cup sour cream
- Sliced jalapeños (optional)

Preparation:

In a skillet, cook the ground meat over medium heat until browned. Add taco seasoning and water as directed on the packet.

In a large bowl, layer lettuce, cooked meat, tomatoes, and cheese.

Top with sour cream and jalapeños if desired.

Balsamic Glazed Brussels Sprouts

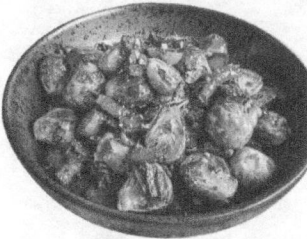

Ingredients:
- 1 pound Brussels sprouts, halved
- 2 tablespoons olive oil

- 1/4 cup balsamic vinegar
- Salt and pepper to taste

Preparation:

Preheat the oven to 400°F (200°C).

Toss Brussels sprouts with olive oil, balsamic vinegar, salt, and pepper.

Spread on a baking sheet and roast for 20-25 minutes, until tender and caramelized.

Chicken and Vegetable Stir-Fry

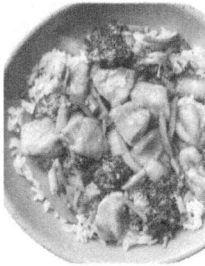

Ingredients:

- 1 pound chicken breast, sliced
- 2 cups mixed vegetables (broccoli, bell peppers, snap peas)
- 3 tablespoons soy sauce (or tamari)

- 1 tablespoon sesame oil
- 1 tablespoon fresh ginger, minced

Preparation:

Heat sesame oil in a large skillet over medium-high heat.

Add chicken and cook until browned, about 5-7 minutes.

Stir in vegetables, ginger, and soy sauce. Cook for an additional 5 minutes until vegetables are tender.

Stuffed Avocado with Tuna

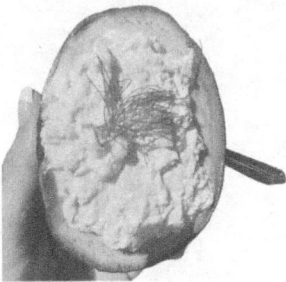

Ingredients:

- 2 ripe avocados, halved and pitted
- 1 can tuna, drained

- 2 tablespoons mayonnaise
- 1 tablespoon Dijon mustard
- Salt and pepper to taste

Preparation:

In a bowl, mix tuna, mayonnaise, mustard, salt, and pepper.

Scoop tuna mixture into avocado halves.

Serve chilled or at room temperature.

Moroccan-Spiced Lamb Chops

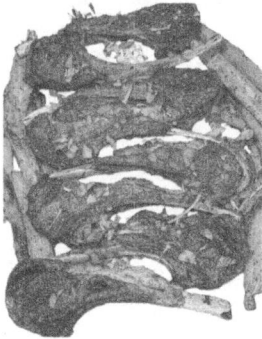

Ingredients:
- 4 lamb chops
- 2 tablespoons olive oil

- 1 tablespoon Moroccan spice blend (cumin, coriander, paprika)
- Salt and pepper to taste

Preparation:
Preheat the grill to medium-high heat.
Rub lamb chops with olive oil, Moroccan spice blend, salt, and pepper.
Grill chops for about 4-5 minutes per side for medium-rare, adjusting time based on thickness.
Serve with a side of roasted vegetables.

These lunch and dinner recipes are designed to be easy, nutritious, and full of flavor, ensuring you stay satisfied while adhering to your low-carb lifestyle. Enjoy exploring these delicious options!

Snacking and Social Eating: Staying on Track

Snacking and social eating can pose challenges, especially when trying to maintain a low-carb lifestyle. However, with a little creativity and planning, you can navigate these situations without sacrificing enjoyment or progress. Embracing smart snacking and making mindful choices during social gatherings will keep you on track and allow you to savor every moment.

First, let's talk about snacking. It's essential to choose snacks that are not only satisfying but also align with your goals. Think about options that provide nourishment without unnecessary carbs. Nuts are a fantastic choice; they're portable, filling, and packed with healthy fats. Consider almonds, walnuts, or pecans as your go-to snacks. Pair them with a piece of cheese for a delightful combination of protein and fat that will keep hunger at bay.

Veggies with dip can also be a winning snack. Crunchy celery, cucumber, and bell peppers dipped in guacamole or a creamy ranch dressing are not only refreshing but also low in carbs. This approach provides you with essential nutrients while keeping you satisfied. Preparing snack bags ahead of time can make it easier to grab a healthy option on the go.

Now, let's turn to social eating. It's common to feel pressure at gatherings, but having a strategy in place can alleviate that anxiety. When you arrive at an event, take a moment to survey the food options available. Look for dishes that are naturally low in carbs, such as salads, cheese platters, or grilled meats. These can often be the foundation of a satisfying meal.

Don't hesitate to ask about ingredients or preparation methods. Many hosts appreciate guests who show interest in the food being served. If the main course includes high-carb items, consider filling your plate with the protein and veggies available. This way, you're enjoying the meal without overindulging in carbs.

If you know you'll be attending a party or gathering, consider bringing a dish of your own. This not only ensures you have a low-carb option but also allows you to share something delicious with others. A creamy spinach dip or a savory zucchini bake can be crowd-pleasers that align with your eating plan. By contributing, you take control of your options while adding variety to the spread.

Mindfulness plays a crucial role in social settings. Enjoy the company around you, engage in conversations, and savor each bite. It's easy to mindlessly snack while chatting, which can lead to consuming more than intended. By being present, you can appreciate the flavors and textures of the food, making you less likely to overeat.

When it comes to beverages, be mindful of your choices. While cocktails and sugary drinks are tempting, opt for sparkling water, herbal teas, or dry wines instead. These options can keep you refreshed without compromising your goals. If you indulge in a drink, choose wisely and balance it with lower-carb food choices.

Lastly, it's important to remember that occasional indulgences are part of life. If you find yourself in a situation where high-carb foods are unavoidable, enjoy them without guilt. The key is moderation. One meal or snack won't derail your progress; it's the overall pattern that matters. Allowing yourself flexibility can make your journey enjoyable and sustainable.

By being proactive and mindful, you can enjoy snacking and social eating while staying aligned with your goals. Embrace the variety of flavors and experiences that come with these moments. With a little planning and a positive mindset, you can navigate any social situation with confidence, enjoying every bite while staying on track.

Chapter 5: Overcoming Challenges and Staying Motivated

Common Mistakes and How to Avoid Them

Embarking on a low-carb journey can be rewarding, but it also comes with its share of challenges. Recognizing common mistakes and knowing how to navigate them can help you maintain your motivation and stay on track. Awareness is the first step toward success, so let's explore some pitfalls and how to overcome them.

One frequent mistake is underestimating portion sizes. It's easy to fall into the trap of thinking that low-carb foods can be consumed in unlimited quantities. Whole foods like nuts and cheese are nutritious, they are also calorie-dense. Paying attention to serving sizes can help you avoid unexpected weight gain. Consider using measuring tools or visual cues to gauge portions until you develop a better understanding of what works for you.

Another common error is neglecting to plan meals and snacks. Without a structured approach, it's easy to grab convenience foods that may not align with your goals. Take time each week to plan your meals, create a grocery list, and prep snacks in advance. This not only ensures that you have healthy options on hand but also minimizes the temptation to reach for higher-carb alternatives during busy moments. Meal prepping can also introduce you to new recipes and flavors, keeping your diet exciting.

Social situations can also present challenges. Many people struggle to navigate gatherings where food is central to the experience. If you find yourself at a party with limited low-carb options, it's easy to feel deprived or overwhelmed. To combat this, plan ahead. Consider eating a healthy snack before you arrive to lessen the temptation to indulge in high-carb foods. Also, don't hesitate to bring your own dish to share. This way, you know there's something you can enjoy that aligns with your eating plan.

Another challenge is emotional eating. Stress, boredom, or sadness can trigger cravings for comfort foods that may not fit within your low-carb framework. Instead of reaching for snacks during these moments, find alternative coping strategies. Engage in activities that lift your spirits, such as going for a walk, practicing mindfulness, or calling a friend. Develop a collection of wholesome coping mechanisms to overcome emotional eating triggers.

Sometimes, individuals may experience fatigue or boredom with their food choices. Eating the same meals repeatedly can lead to a lack of motivation. To counteract this, explore new recipes and ingredients regularly. Experimenting with different cooking techniques or cuisines can add excitement to your meals. Consider joining online communities or forums where you can exchange ideas and inspiration with others on a similar journey.

Another hurdle can be the misconception that you must be perfect. Many people expect themselves to stick rigidly to their plan, leading to feelings of guilt or failure when they stray. It's crucial to understand that slip-ups are part of the process. Rather than focusing on perfection, embrace progress. If you indulge occasionally, don't dwell on it. Reflect on what you learned and move forward with renewed determination.

Finally, track your progress in a way that motivates you. Whether it's through journaling, taking progress photos, or celebrating non-scale victories, find what inspires you. Recognizing your achievements, no matter how small, can help maintain your momentum and remind you of your journey's positive aspects.

Overcoming challenges and staying motivated on a low-carb journey requires self-awareness, planning, and flexibility. By understanding common mistakes and implementing strategies to avoid them, you can navigate your path with confidence. Embrace the journey, savor the successes, and remember that every step you take brings you closer to your goals. With the right mindset and tools, you can thrive in your low-carb lifestyle, enjoying the process as much as the results.

Staying Motivated: Mindset Shifts for Success

Staying motivated on your low-carb journey often comes down to cultivating the right mindset. Shifting your perspective can make a significant difference in how you approach challenges and celebrate successes. Embracing these mindset changes will help you navigate your path with enthusiasm and resilience.

First, focus on progress rather than perfection. It's easy to get caught up in the desire to adhere strictly to your plan, but the reality is that setbacks can happen. Rather than viewing a slip-up as a failure, consider it a learning opportunity. Every experience teaches you something valuable about your habits and preferences. Celebrate the small victories along the way, like choosing a healthy snack or preparing a new recipe. This positive reinforcement can fuel your motivation and help you stay committed.

Another essential mindset shift involves self-compassion. Be kind to yourself during this journey. Understand that making lifestyle changes is challenging, and it's natural to have ups and downs. Replace self-criticism with self-encouragement and become your own strongest ally. Acknowledge your efforts and remind yourself that every step, no matter how small, contributes to your overall progress. This self-love can boost your confidence and encourage you to keep going, even when things get tough.

Visualizing your goals can also be a powerful tool. Take a moment to imagine how you will feel once you achieve your desired outcomes. Picture yourself with increased energy, enjoying activities you love, and feeling confident in your skin. Creating a vision board can help solidify these images, serving as a daily reminder of what you're working toward. When you encounter obstacles, this visualization can reignite your passion and remind you why you started.

Surrounding yourself with a supportive community is another crucial aspect of staying motivated. Connect with others who share similar aspirations and struggles for mutual understanding and motivation. Whether through social media groups, local meetups, or online forums, finding a support system can provide encouragement and inspiration. Sharing your experiences and hearing from others can help you feel less isolated and more empowered. Plus, you'll discover new tips and strategies that can enhance your journey.

Additionally, embrace the concept of experimentation. Treat your low-carb journey as an adventure rather than a rigid program. Try new recipes, explore different ingredients, and discover what works best for your body and taste preferences. This playful approach can make the process enjoyable and help you avoid monotony. When you view your meals as opportunities for creativity, you'll likely find greater satisfaction and motivation.

Mindfulness also plays a significant role in maintaining motivation. Practicing mindfulness can help you become more aware of your cravings and emotional triggers. When you feel the urge to snack or indulge, take a moment to pause and reflect on what you truly need. Are you hungry, or is it boredom or stress? By recognizing these feelings, you can make more conscious choices that align with your goals.

Finally, remember that this journey is uniquely yours. Avoid comparing your progress to others, as everyone has different experiences and timelines. Focus on your own path and celebrate your individual achievements. By embracing your journey and honoring your choices, you'll cultivate a sense of ownership that can drive your motivation.

Staying motivated is about fostering a mindset that empowers you. By shifting your focus to progress, practicing self-compassion, visualizing your goals, and engaging with a supportive community, you can navigate challenges with confidence. Embrace experimentation, practice mindfulness, and remember that your journey is personal. With the right mindset, you can thrive on your low-carb path, finding joy in each step you take.

Maintaining Progress: Overcoming Plateaus

Sometimes, when everything seems to be going well, progress slows or stalls unexpectedly. This is a common experience and can happen for many reasons. It might feel frustrating, but these moments don't mean failure. They are just an opportunity to reassess, adjust, and keep moving forward. Plateaus are a normal part of any transformation and often signal that it's time to fine-tune your approach.

One of the reasons this can happen is that your body has adapted to the changes. When you first begin making adjustments to your lifestyle, it's a bit of a shock to the system, causing rapid changes. But over time, your body gets used to the new routine, and the progress you were seeing slows down. This doesn't mean you've reached your destination, but that your journey needs a little change of direction.

What worked at the beginning may not work as effectively now, and this is where flexibility becomes key. Small changes can have a significant impact. It could be as simple as adjusting your intake slightly or changing up your routine to challenge your body in different ways. The idea is to stay consistent but introduce new elements that prevent stagnation.

Another reason for hitting a standstill is stress, whether from daily life or from putting too much pressure on yourself to see quick results. Stress can slow progress without you even realizing it. When this happens, it's important to take a step back and focus on balance. This isn't just about what you eat or how you move, but also how you take care of your mind. Adding relaxation techniques or just allowing yourself to rest more can work wonders for breaking through that barrier.

Staying positive is also critical during this time. It's easy to get discouraged when progress isn't as fast as expected, but staying focused on the long-term goal is essential. Sometimes the changes happening are not immediately visible. Remember that internal shifts can be just as important as the outward ones. This period is about staying patient and persistent, knowing that progress, no matter how slow, is still progress.

Another way to move forward is to revisit your original plan and see if any old habits have crept back in unnoticed. Over time, it's easy to let little things slide, and those small details can add up. This is a perfect time to refocus and make sure you're sticking to the principles that have been effective so far.

Also, keep in mind that your body's needs can change as you go along. What felt satisfying in the beginning might need to be adjusted to suit your evolving needs. Listening to what your body is telling you is essential, and learning to respond with small tweaks will help you continue to see progress.

The key to moving beyond a plateau is persistence. It's about trusting the process and being willing to make adjustments. Keep experimenting with small changes, stay consistent, and above all, remember that plateaus are temporary. The critical element is determination; never give up. Keep going, and you'll break through.

Conclusion and Next Steps

As you reach the conclusion of your journey, take a moment to reflect on the transformative path you've embarked upon. Adopting a low-carb lifestyle is not merely a dietary change; it's a commitment to nurturing your body and embracing a healthier, more vibrant life. The strategies and insights you've gained throughout this book are designed to empower you, making it easier to navigate your daily choices and cultivate habits that support your goals.

Every step you've taken—whether it's stocking your pantry with nourishing foods, learning to appreciate the flavors of whole ingredients, or overcoming the challenges of breaking free from sugar and processed foods—contributes to a greater sense of well-being. Remember, this journey is unique to you. Celebrate your progress, no matter how small, and acknowledge the strength it takes to make lasting changes.

In the initial phases, you may have experienced challenges, but those moments are invaluable learning opportunities. As your body adapts and your taste buds evolve, you'll discover newfound satisfaction in foods that fuel your energy and support your health. The keys to success lie not only in understanding what to eat but also in developing a positive relationship with food that prioritizes your well-being.

As you continue this journey, keep exploring. The world of low-carb eating is filled with endless possibilities, from creative recipes to diverse cuisines. Allow yourself the freedom to experiment in the kitchen, discover new flavors, and share your culinary creations with others. Cooking can become a source of joy and creativity, rather than a mundane task, inviting you to savor each meal fully.

Moreover, don't hesitate to seek support from others. Whether through communities, friends, or family, sharing your experiences can foster motivation and accountability. Surrounding yourself with like-minded individuals can help you stay inspired and engaged in your journey toward better health.

Looking ahead, remember that this lifestyle is about more than just weight loss; it's about nourishing your body and embracing a holistic approach to wellness. As you move forward, focus on how you feel—both physically and emotionally. The energy, clarity, and confidence that come from fueling your body with nutritious, low-carb foods are invaluable gifts that extend far beyond the scale.

Your journey doesn't end here. Each day presents new opportunities to reinforce your commitment to a healthier lifestyle. Embrace the knowledge you've gained, stay curious, and continue to learn about your body's needs. With patience and perseverance, you'll build a sustainable lifestyle that serves you for years to come.

As you take these final steps, carry with you the belief that you have the power to transform your body and change your life. This journey is yours, and every choice you make is a step toward achieving your goals. Celebrate your commitment, enjoy the process, and savor the delicious, nourishing foods that support your journey to a healthier, happier you. Your best self awaits, and this is just the beginning.

Resources for Ongoing Support and Education

As you continue on your journey toward a healthier lifestyle, having access to the right resources can make a significant difference. The world of low-carb nutrition is dynamic, with new information, recipes, and support systems emerging regularly. Below are some valuable resources that can provide ongoing support, education, and inspiration as you progress on your path.

Online Communities and Support Groups

Engaging with others on a similar journey can be incredibly motivating. Online communities provide a space to share experiences, seek advice, and celebrate successes. Websites like **Reddit** host subreddits such as **r/Atkins** and **r/loseit**, offering forums where members share tips, recipes, and encouragement. These platforms allow for open discussions, giving you access to a wealth of knowledge and experience from people who have successfully navigated the same path. Facebook groups dedicated to low-carb lifestyles can connect you with thousands of like-minded individuals who share insights, meal ideas, and support. Look for groups with active engagement and a positive atmosphere, as these environments can foster a sense of camaraderie and accountability.

Apps for Tracking and Meal Planning

In this digital age, several apps can assist you in tracking your food intake and planning meals effectively. **MyFitnessPal** allows you to log your meals and monitor your macronutrients, helping you stay accountable. Its extensive food database makes it easy to find and input meals, providing valuable insights into your dietary habits. **Carb**

Manager is another excellent app specifically designed for those following low-carb diets, offering features that allow you to track your carbohydrate intake easily. This app includes a barcode scanner for quick entry and a library of low-carb recipes.

For meal planning, apps like **Mealime** and **Paprika** can help you create customized meal plans that align with your dietary goals. These apps allow you to generate shopping lists based on your selected recipes, making grocery shopping more efficient. Additionally, **Yummly** provides personalized recipe recommendations based on your preferences and dietary restrictions, allowing you to discover new meals that excite your palate.

Educational Websites and Blogs

Staying informed is essential for long-term success. Websites like **Diet Doctor** offer extensive resources, including articles, meal plans, and recipes tailored to low-carb lifestyles. The site features a variety of content, from beginner guides to in-depth analyses of the latest research on low-carb diets. **Ruled.me** is another popular blog that provides practical tips, delicious recipes, and personal stories from individuals who have successfully transitioned to low-carb eating. The testimonials shared on this platform can inspire and motivate you as you navigate your journey.

For evidence-based information, the **American Journal of Clinical Nutrition** and **Nutrition & Metabolism** publish research studies that can deepen your understanding of low-carb diets and their effects on health. Following reputable nutritionists and dietitians on social media platforms like Instagram or Twitter can also keep you updated with the latest insights, tips, and research findings.

Podcasts and YouTube Channels

Podcasts can be a great way to absorb information while on the go. Shows like **"The Keto Diet Podcast"** and **"The Low Carb MD Podcast"** feature interviews with experts and discussions about various aspects of low-carb living. These podcasts often include success stories, allowing you to learn from others' experiences and gather practical advice.

On platforms like YouTube, channels such as **"Keto Connect"** and **"Headbanger's Kitchen"** offer visual cooking demonstrations, meal prep tips, and insights into low-carb lifestyles. YouTube is a treasure trove of recipe ideas, cooking techniques, and meal inspiration, making it easy to find content that resonates with your personal taste. Channels like **"Thomas DeLauer"** provide informative videos on the science behind low-carb eating, intermittent fasting, and healthy lifestyle changes.

Local Resources

Don't overlook local resources that can support your journey. Consider seeking out nutritionists or dietitians who specialize in low-carb diets. Many offer personalized consultations to help you tailor your dietary approach to your individual needs. These professionals can provide valuable insights into meal planning, food choices, and overcoming any obstacles you may face. Additionally, local health food stores and farmers' markets often provide fresh, low-carb options and can be great places to meet others interested in healthy eating. Building relationships with local vendors can also give you access to high-quality, fresh produce and other low-carb staples.

Meal Delivery Services

If you find meal prep challenging, consider meal delivery services that cater to low-carb diets. Companies like **Snap Kitchen** and **Trifecta** provide pre-prepared meals that align with low-carb principles, making it easier to stay on track without the hassle of cooking. These services often offer a variety of options, allowing you to select meals that fit your taste preferences and dietary needs.

For those looking for more variety, consider services like **Green Chef** or **HelloFresh,** which offer low-carb meal kits that come with pre-measured ingredients and easy-to-follow recipes. This approach simplifies the cooking process and encourages you to try new dishes that you might not have prepared otherwise.

Continuing Education

To deepen your understanding of nutrition and health, consider enrolling in online courses or workshops. Websites like **Coursera** and **Udemy** offer courses on nutrition, healthy cooking, and wellness that can enhance your knowledge and skills. These courses often feature expert instructors and cover a range of topics, allowing you to explore various aspects of low-carb living at your own pace.

Additionally, look for local workshops or seminars focused on nutrition and healthy eating. Many community centers and health organizations offer classes that provide hands-on experience in meal preparation and nutrition education. Participating in these events can foster connections with others interested in similar lifestyle changes and provide a supportive community.

Blogs and Social Media Influencers

As you continue your journey, consider following prominent bloggers and social media influencers who specialize in low-carb living. Figures like **Maria Emmerich** and **Keto Adapted** share recipes, tips, and personal stories that can keep you motivated. Social media platforms like Instagram are ideal for discovering meal ideas and inspiration from fellow low-carb enthusiasts. Look for hashtags like **#low carb** or **#keto** to find posts from individuals who share their culinary creations and success stories.

ADDED BONUS: 30-DAYS MEAL PLAN

Week 1: Induction Phase (Days 1-7)

DAY 1:

Breakfast: Scrambled eggs with spinach and avocado

Lunch: Grilled chicken breast with roasted vegetables

Dinner: Baked salmon with cauliflower rice

Snacks: Raw veggies with hummus, cheese sticks

DAY 2:

Breakfast: Atkins Diet shake with almond milk and berries

Lunch: Turkey lettuce wraps with avocado and tomato

Dinner: Grilled pork chop with roasted broccoli

Snacks: Hard-boiled eggs, mozzarella cheese balls

DAY 3:

Breakfast: Omelette with mushrooms and feta cheese

Lunch: Chicken Caesar salad

Dinner: Beef stir-fry with vegetables and cauliflower rice

Snacks: Cottage cheese cups, celery sticks with almond butter

DAY 4:

Breakfast: Greek yogurt with berries and chopped nuts

Lunch: Turkey and avocado wrap with lettuce

Dinner: Baked chicken thighs with roasted asparagus

Snacks: Protein bars, raw veggies with hummus

DAY 5:

Breakfast: Avocado toast with scrambled eggs

Lunch: Grilled chicken breast with mixed greens salad

Dinner: Pork tenderloin with roasted Brussels sprouts
Snacks: Mozzarella cheese sticks, Atkins Diet shake

DAY 6:

Breakfast: Smoothie bowl with protein powder and almond milk
Lunch: Turkey and cheese sandwich on low-carb bread
Dinner: Grilled shrimp with zucchini noodles
Snacks: Hard-boiled eggs, cherry tomatoes

DAY 7:

Breakfast: Omelette with vegetables and feta cheese
Lunch: Chicken breast with roasted vegetables
Dinner: Steak with sautéed asparagus and a side salad
Snacks: Greek yogurt with berries, chopped nuts

Week 2: Ongoing Weight Loss (OWL) Phase (Days 8-14)

DAY 8:

Breakfast: Scrambled eggs with chorizo and avocado

Lunch: Spinach salad with grilled chicken, avocado, and olive oil

Dinner: Grilled pork chop with roasted broccoli

Snacks: Raw veggies with hummus, cheese sticks

DAY 9:

Breakfast: Atkins Diet shake with almond milk and berries

Lunch: Chicken Caesar salad

Dinner: Beef stir-fry with vegetables and cauliflower rice

Snacks: Cottage cheese cups, celery sticks with almond butter

DAY 10:

Breakfast: Greek yogurt with berries and chopped nuts

Lunch: Turkey and avocado wrap with lettuce

Dinner: Baked chicken thighs with roasted asparagus

Snacks: Protein bars, raw veggies with hummus

DAY 11:

Breakfast: Deviled eggs with cucumber slices

Lunch: Grilled chicken breast with mixed greens salad

Dinner: Grilled pork tenderloin with sautéed zucchini and mushrooms

Snacks: Mozzarella cheese sticks, Atkins Diet shake

DAY 12:

Breakfast: Smoothie bowl with protein powder and almond milk

Lunch: Turkey and cheese sandwich on low-carb bread

Dinner: Grilled shrimp with zucchini noodles

Snacks: Hard-boiled eggs, cherry tomatoes

DAY 13:

Breakfast: Omelette with vegetables and feta cheese

Lunch: Caesar salad with grilled chicken (no croutons)

Dinner: Pan-seared cod with sautéed spinach

Snacks: Greek yogurt with berries, chopped nuts

DAY 14:

Breakfast: Scrambled eggs with spinach and avocado

Lunch: Turkey lettuce wraps with avocado and tomato

Dinner: Grilled pork chop with roasted broccoli

Snacks: Raw veggies with hummus, cheese sticks

Week 3: Pre-Maintenance Phase (Days 15-21)

DAY 15:
Breakfast: Atkins Diet shake with almond milk and berries
Lunch:Tuna salad with mayo, olives, and cucumbers
Dinner: Grilled chicken thighs with sautéed green beans
Snacks: Cottage cheese cups, celery sticks with almond butter

DAY 16:
Breakfast: Greek yogurt with berries and chopped nuts
Lunch: Turkey and avocado wrap with lettuce
Dinner: Baked chicken thighs with roasted asparagus
Snacks: Protein bars, raw veggies with hummus

DAY 17:

Breakfast: Omelet with mushrooms, cheese, and tomatoes

Lunch: Egg salad lettuce wraps

Dinner: Baked cod with a side of cauliflower mash

Snacks: String cheese with cucumber slices

DAY 18:

Breakfast: Smoothie bowl with protein powder and almond milk

Lunch: Turkey and cheese sandwich on low-carb bread

Dinner: Grilled shrimp with zucchini noodles

Snacks: Hard-boiled eggs, cherry tomatoes

DAY 19:

Breakfast: Omelette with vegetables and feta cheese

Lunch: Chicken breast with roasted vegetables

Dinner: Baked salmon with cauliflower rice

Snacks: Greek yogurt with berries, chopped nuts

DAY 20:

Breakfast: Scrambled eggs with spinach and avocado

Lunch: Turkey lettuce wraps with avocado and tomato

Dinner: Grilled pork chop with roasted broccoli

Snacks: Raw veggies with hummus, cheese sticks

DAY 21:

Breakfast: Atkins Diet shake with almond milk and berries

Lunch: Chicken Caesar salad

Dinner: Grilled lamb chops with a cucumber and feta salad

Snacks: Cottage cheese cups, celery sticks with almond butter

Week 4: Maintenance Phase (Days 22–30)

DAY 22:
Breakfast: Hard-boiled eggs with turkey slices and avocado
Lunch: Turkey lettuce wraps with cheese and mayo
Dinner: Grilled pork chops with roasted Brussels sprouts
Snacks: Mozzarella cheese sticks, Atkins Diet shake

DAY 23:
Breakfast: Smoothie bowl with protein powder and almond milk
Lunch: Turkey and cheese sandwich on low-carb bread
Dinner: Grilled shrimp with zucchini noodles
Snacks: Hard-boiled eggs, cherry tomatoes

DAY 24:

Breakfast: Poached eggs with smoked salmon and cream cheese

Lunch: Cobb salad (lettuce, bacon, avocado, chicken, boiled egg, and blue cheese)

Dinner: Grilled steak with roasted zucchini

Snacks: Greek yogurt with berries, chopped nuts

DAY 25:

Breakfast: Scrambled eggs with spinach and avocado

Lunch: Turkey lettuce wraps with avocado and tomato

Dinner: Grilled pork chop with roasted broccoli

Snacks: Raw veggies with hummus, cheese sticks

DAY 26:

Breakfast: Atkins Diet shake with almond milk and berries

Lunch: Shrimp salad with avocado and mixed greens

Dinner: Grilled pork tenderloin with a side of roasted cauliflower

Snacks: Cottage cheese cups, celery sticks with almond butter

DAY 27:

Breakfast: Avocado toast with scrambled eggs

Lunch: Grilled chicken breast with mixed greens salad

Dinner: Pork tenderloin with roasted Brussels sprouts

Snacks: Mozzarella cheese sticks, Atkins Diet shake

DAY 28:

Breakfast: Smoothie bowl with protein powder and almond milk

Lunch: Turkey and cheese sandwich on low-carb bread

Dinner: Grilled shrimp with zucchini noodles

Snacks: Hard-boiled eggs, cherry tomatoes

DAY 29:

Breakfast: Omelette with vegetables and feta cheese

Lunch: Chicken breast with roasted vegetables

Dinner: Baked salmon with broccoli and garlic butter

Snacks: Greek yogurt with berries, chopped nuts

DAY 30:

Breakfast: Scrambled eggs with spinach and avocado

Lunch: Turkey lettuce wraps with avocado and tomato

Dinner: Grilled steak with roasted Brussels sprouts

Snacks: Raw veggies with hummus, cheese sticks

Macro Breakdown:

Protein: 150-200g/day

Fat: 50-70g/day

Carbohydrates: 20-50g/day (depending on phase)

Tips and Variations:

Drink at least 8 glasses of water per day.
Perform physical activity, such as walking or light exercise.
Swap protein sources and vegetables to avoid repetition.
Adjust portion sizes based on individual calorie needs.

WEEKLY MEAL PLANNER (week 1-4)

WEEKLY —

Meal Planner

Week of:

Monday	Tuesday	Wednesday
BREAKFAST	BREAKFAST	BREAKFAST
LUNCH	LUNCH	LUNCH
DINNER	DINNER	DINNER
SNACK	SNACK	SNACK

Thursday	Friday	Saturday
BREAKFAST	BREAKFAST	BREAKFAST
LUNCH	LUNCH	LUNCH
DINNER	DINNER	DINNER
SNACK	SNACK	SNACK

Sunday	NOTES:
BREAKFAST	
LUNCH	
DINNER	
SNACK	

Meal Planner

Week of: _____

Monday		Tuesday		Wednesday
BREAKFAST		BREAKFAST		BREAKFAST
LUNCH		LUNCH		LUNCH
DINNER		DINNER		DINNER
SNACK		SNACK		SNACK

Thursday		Friday		Saturday
BREAKFAST		BREAKFAST		BREAKFAST
LUNCH		LUNCH		LUNCH
DINNER		DINNER		DINNER
SNACK		SNACK		SNACK

Sunday	NOTES:
BREAKFAST	
LUNCH	
DINNER	
SNACK	

Meal Planner

Week of: _____

Monday		Tuesday		Wednesday
BREAKFAST		BREAKFAST		BREAKFAST
LUNCH		LUNCH		LUNCH
DINNER		DINNER		DINNER
SNACK		SNACK		SNACK

Thursday		Friday		Saturday
BREAKFAST		BREAKFAST		BREAKFAST
LUNCH		LUNCH		LUNCH
DINNER		DINNER		DINNER
SNACK		SNACK		SNACK

Sunday	NOTES:
BREAKFAST	
LUNCH	
DINNER	
SNACK	

Meal Planner

Week of: _____

Monday		Tuesday		Wednesday
BREAKFAST		BREAKFAST		BREAKFAST
LUNCH		LUNCH		LUNCH
DINNER		DINNER		DINNER
SNACK		SNACK		SNACK

Thursday		Friday		Saturday
BREAKFAST		BREAKFAST		BREAKFAST
LUNCH		LUNCH		LUNCH
DINNER		DINNER		DINNER
SNACK		SNACK		SNACK

Sunday	NOTES:
BREAKFAST	
LUNCH	
DINNER	
SNACK	

Additional Notes

Notes

Made in United States
Cleveland, OH
04 March 2025